FOOTNOTES

FOOTNOTES

A Life Without Limits

LENA MARIA KLINGVALL

Health Communications, Inc.
Deerfield Beach, Florida

www.hci-online.com

Library of Congress Cataloging-in-Publication Data

Klingvall, Lena Maria.
   Footnotes : a life without limits / Lena Maria.
      p.   cm
   ISBN 1-55874-911-X (pbk.)
   1. Klingvall, Lena Maria.   2. Physically handicapped—
Biography.   3. Extremities (Anatomy)—Abnormalities.
4. Musculoskeletal system—Abnormalities.   I. Title.

   RD775.K565 2001
   362.4'3'092—dc21
   [B]

                                                      2001020421

Publisher: Health Communications, Inc.
               3201 S.W. 15th Street
               Deerfield Beach, FL 33442-8190

Cover and inside design by Lawna Patterson Oldfield
Inside book formatting by Dawn Grove

Contents

Preface

When I meet new people, they often reach out a hand to greet me but only receive a "hi" back. Some soon regain their composure, withdraw their hands and greet me with a smile or give me a hug. Other people become incredibly self-conscious and don't know how to get out of this situation, which they have experienced as extremely embarrassing.

Sometimes such people come up to me several years later to ask me if I can remember how embarrassing it was when I met them for the first time because they had greeted me in the wrong way. Fortunately, I seldom remember such occasions. I cannot shake hands with people, because I do not have any arms.

People react very differently to me and my disability. A few years ago a lady came up to me to give me some money because she felt so sorry for me.

When I was a child and my parents and I were having a meal in a restaurant, my eating habits inspired the children at an adjacent table so much that they pulled in their arms under their pullovers, put up their feet on the table and tried to eat exactly the way I was eating. I thought their reaction was wonderful, even though it embarrassed their parents.

One advantage in not having arms and hands in never having to lose rings or gloves. Once when I was little and had been playing at a classmate's, my dad came to pick me up. I put my hat, jacket and shoes on while my friend's mother was running around excitedly looking for gloves for me to use.

"They won't be needed," said my dad.

"But it is so cold. Of course she must have some gloves," said the mother.

However, soon she realized that perhaps they would not be needed after all. . . .

And when I was in the sixth school year, I had an assistant who was so kind to me that she bought me a Christmas present. The day before Christmas Eve she realized her mistake: She had bought me a ring! She hurried back to the shop and bought me a necklace instead.

On another occasion, I remember that I was wearing a bracelet on my right ankle. It was very unusual to wear ankle bracelets at that time, so a classmate came up to me and asked why I was wearing the bracelet around my ankle instead of around my wrist.

"It is a little difficult for me," I said, and her cheeks reddened.

Episodes like this one amuse me a great deal. I actually enjoy seeing people making faux pas, more or less. Not because I really want them to feel embarrassed, but because it shows that they have not noticed, or do not think about, the fact that I am disabled. It is wonderful when people who have known me for some time see me and my disability in the same way as I do. Usually they forget my disability.

In this book, I want to tell you a little about myself and the things that have contributed to my being the person I am today. At the time of writing, there is still some time left until I turn thirty, but I have already experienced much which has been enjoyable—and quite a lot of things which probably nobody could have imagined when I was born.

Naturally, my disability has influenced me in more ways than one, but I have been influenced just as much by singing and music and all that has come into my life from these gifts. I have also been influenced by my successes in swimming, my family and friends, and my faith in God. These are the things that I want to tell you about in this book.

Writing a book has been quite a new experience for me. I would never have managed to do it had it not been for the help I have received from Inger Lundin. I want to take this opportunity to give her a big thank you!

It would be pretentious to call my story "memoirs," even though this might be correct. It is quite simply a few notes and a few comments on life as far as I have lived it.

They are my footnotes.

1

"She Will Need a Home Anyway"

N obody said anything.

Immediately after I was born, the midwife took hold of me, turned around, put me in a towel and carried me into an adjacent room. Everything went so quickly. The delivery room was full of people. There was my mother, of course, and the midwife, and my dad was at my mum's side, and then there was a crowd of doctors and nurses who were doing their routine rounds. But everything went so extremely quickly. All the visitors were herded out, my dad was told to go and sit in the waiting room, and my mum was left alone. Nobody said anything.

It was September twenty-eighth at eight o'clock in the morning, and I had just seen the light of day.

Nobody had thought that I would not look like everybody else. Nobody could have imagined that I would be "malformed." The pregnancy had been normal in every way as far as it had been possible to see. This, of course, was before fetus diagnosis and ultrasound had become common features of prenatal care, so nothing abnormal had been detected.

The delivery had been hard for my mother, Anna. When her water broke in the afternoon of September twenty-sixth, she went into the maternity wing of the Jönköping Hospital. My father, Rolf, had just barely been given leave from his month's military service in Uddevalla. My mother was relieved and happy that he came, because the labor was a very long and drawn-out one. One night, one day, and then another night, but then, after thirty-four hours of hard work for my mother, I was born.

I was 48 centimeters (or just over 19 inches) long but weighed only 2,400 grams (5 pounds, 6 ounces). Where there should have been arms was nothing. Where my shoulders finished were just two small stumps. My right leg looked quite normal, but my left leg was only about half the size of my right one. My left foot stuck up almost vertically and was lying alongside my leg. Furthermore, my face was blue when I was born. Might there be inner injuries as well? Was I going to die, or would I survive? The hospital staff did not know. This is why they took me to another room.

To start with, Mum and Dad understood nothing. Because I was their first child, they had no idea what kind of routine could be expected after a delivery, whether at Jönköping's hospital or anywhere else. So my being taken to another room and my dad being shown into the waiting room were things they thought were commonplace.

After an hour or more, a doctor came in and explained about the situation and my handicap, first to Dad in the waiting room, and then to Mum. He told them what had happened and tried to do so as calmly and matter-of-factly as possible. He offered them tranquilizers. The doctor could not be sure that I would survive until they had checked to see if my internal organs were damaged as well. He informed them that if I survived there was the possibility of them having to leave such a severely disabled child in an institution.

My parents were about to make a difficult decision.

"You will have to consider caring for her for at least twenty years if you do it yourselves," said the doctor.

My mum was so exhausted after the delivery and so dulled by the laughing gas she had been given as a pain-reliever that, to start with, she didn't understand how serious the situation was. It was not until my dad came in and explained it again to her that she understood. But they still had not seen me.

The next three days were very heavy for them. What should have been a message of joy to the relatives became a message of sorrow instead. Dad rang around to all our relatives. My maternal grandpa and grandma and my mother's sister, Brita, came to the hospital and sat on Mum's bed crying. Would I survive? How would my life be? How did I actually look?

And what did God mean? Both my parents were Christians, active members of the local Covenant church, who had a strong faith in God, but now many thoughts flew through their minds. When Dad came home from the hospital the first time after the delivery he fell down on his knees by his bed and prayed to God. I know he had a lot of questions to ask God, and he told God that now he would have to take care of the future.

My parents tried to comfort each other. Quite soon my mum had to start pumping milk from her breasts. I was fed this milk in the ward where I was, and this was a step forward in itself. I was able to keep the food down, and the machinery inside was working.

After three days, they were at last allowed to see me. My mother, who was still weak after the delivery, was pushed in a wheelchair through the culvert to the ward where I was.

They were a bit nervous. From the doctors' description of my handicap they did not know quite what to expect.

They looked at me through the glass pane. There I

was lying in a cot, all five pounds, six ounces of Lena Johansson, pursing my mouth and looking as healthy and thriving as anybody else. They felt that I looked so fine, much better than they had ever been led to expect!

I do not know for sure, but I think it was just about then that my parents made up their minds that they would take care of me and bring me up themselves. It was not something to be taken for granted. There were many who spoke for institutional care, and both my parents realized quite clearly that such a severe disability as mine would mean an enormous amount of work.

I think it was my dad's comment that sealed the decision:

"Arms or no arms, she will need a home anyway."

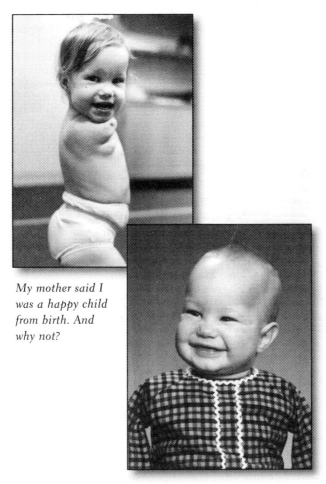

My mother said I was a happy child from birth. And why not?

Me, aged two

|2

With the Bottle
Around My
Big Toe

W hy?
      Many people believe that I suffered damage because of thalidomide, the tranquilizer with side effects that caused a fetus not to develop normally, resulting in misshapen arms and legs. But this was not the reason in my case. When my mother was expecting me, this particular medicine had already been forbidden. All the debate in the press and television had made my mother extra careful so that she did not take any medicines whatsoever during her pregnancy.

For a long time, the doctors were puzzled, but now

they believe that I am one of a very small number of people who are born even though we actually "ought not to be." When a fetus starts to develop wrongly, the mother's body normally rejects it. However, in a few very rare cases the body's natural rejection system does not work, and the pregnancy continues to completion. That's why I was born.

A great number of investigations were done at the hospital, but after two weeks I was allowed to come home. My mother is of the opinion that I had a happy nature from the beginning, and this is probably right. Why shouldn't I have been happy? I could hardly have known that I was lacking certain body parts, and I did not hurt anywhere. I learned faster than most to roll around from my back onto my tummy in bed, since no arms were in the way. Then I lay on my tummy, lifting my curious head and looking around over the side of the crib. My neck muscles were quite something!

It was of course very natural that I used my legs a lot. If you observe babies for a while, you will find that they grip with both hands and feet. When other babies had to learn to use their hands more and more, I started to develop my footwork.

After five weeks, I started to play with the pacifier with my foot, and quite soon I could also suck on my big toe whenever I wanted to. After a while, my mum discovered that if there was a rubber band around the milk bottle and this was attached around my big toe I could drink my milk completely by myself. I liked that. I developed and learned new things, even though I may not have learned them at the same speed as the average child.

For my mum, the first year of my life was particularly heavy. She was the one who took care of me the most and allowed me to become accustomed to new surroundings. My dad hesitated to do this, and it is probably fairly easy to understand why. Wherever Mum took me, she was met with stares, curious comments and stupid questions.

When I was due to be taken to the well-baby clinic for my first postnatal checkup, Mum asked for an appointment when there would not be any other parents and children there. She was given one, and nobody else was there. However, the district nurse had a long talk with Mum about the importance of coming in the future at times when there would be other mothers there with their children. The nurse said it was important that other people got to see that they shouldn't assume that everybody should look the same.

Before we were ushered in to see the doctor the nurse had been asked to inform him concerning my anatomy so that he would be a little prepared. His back was turned towards us when we first entered the room, and my mum was asked to undress me. Then he turned around and was probably quite shocked.

"Oh dear! How terrible!"

Mum burst into tears. The nurse had forgotten to inform the doctor.

She found it stressful all the time to have to tell new acquaintances about my disability. She really wanted to feel proud of me, but it was not always a matter of course. It seldom happened that somebody asked those ordinary questions that every mother is so happy to answer:

Did I sleep well at night?

Did I eat well?

Was I gaining weight?

What developments had I reached?

Well, I knew, for example, several tricks that I could do with my right foot, and I had gradually learned to grip objects with my shoulder and chin, but it was easy for people around me to concentrate only on that which did not work.

For instance, the problem with my left foot. It was seriously deformed and was lying quite close to my leg. The foot stuck straight up. To start with it did not occur to anyone that it might be possible to improve the situation. However, one person saw the possibilities — Lars-Göran Ottosson, the registrar in charge of the physiotherapy clinic in Jönköping. Thanks to him I was fitted with a metal splint for my left foot which helped straighten it out to the normal position.

The doctors also came to see how they could help me get a better grip with my chin. I had an operation in which one of my ribs was moved up and positioned at exactly the same height as my shoulder. This enabled me to obtain a much larger grip area against my right shoulder. This operation was done when I was only one year old, but that innovation is still helping me enormously.

It took a while before I learned how to move about. Initially, before I learned to sit up, I used to roll around in order to move forward. Next I developed the trick of travelling on my bottom by pushing myself forward with the help of my right leg.

When I was about three years old, I received my first prosthetic limb for my left leg. By this time my left foot had had time to shape itself with the help of the metal splint and a bandage, and it was now turned into a fairly normal position. But learning to walk for the first time was very, very difficult. It took time.

My parents got the idea that they could use a harness when they taught me to walk. Since I had no arms or hands there was nothing for them to hold on to. They used the kind of harness that is normally used in carriages to keep babies from falling out. They also attached an additional leather strap between my legs so that the harness would not glide up above my head, and it would give support. Yet another, longer, leather strap was attached on the back which helped them to hold on to me and hold me up when I was about to fall.

In other words, it was "trial and error" all the time, but it went a little better each day until finally I could walk without help. I had very poor balance, so I often fell over. On many occasions I fell headlong. My chin had to take a lot of bashing. On Christmas Eve one year, I slipped down an icy flight of stone stairs and hit my chin so badly that I had to be taken to the emergency room of the hospital to be stitched up.

But the fact remained—I was walking!

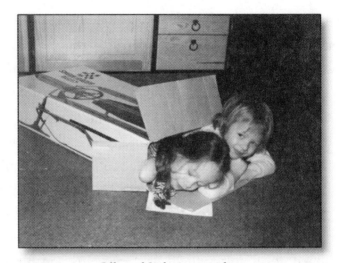

Olle and I playing together

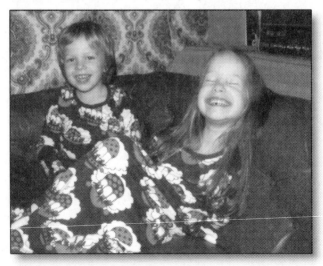

Sometimes my brother and I dressed alike.

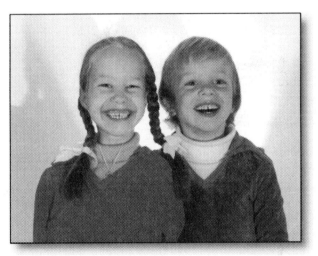

This picture was taken when I was nine years old.
My brother Olle was eight.

3

Helping
Without
Hindering

My brother Olle was born when I was only just over a year old. My parents had been advised to try and have another baby as soon as possible after my birth in order to be able to compare my development with another child of approximately the same age. The medical profession felt there would be only a minimal risk that he would also be afflicted with a similar handicap, and sure enough, he came out with both arms and legs.

When I was two years old, our family bought a farm and we became "country folks." The farm was called Nydala. It was situated in Klerebo in Bankeryd, about nine miles northwest of Jönköping and was a secluded and idyllic place with a lovely view over a lake. We actually lived in the province of Västergötland, even though we lived near Jönköping. We fetched our mail in the province of Småland, though, as the border went right between our house and our mailbox down by the main road.

Mum was at home full-time with me and Olle for my first ten years. She had had time to work as a physiotherapist for a while before having children and made good use of her education also as a full-time mum.

My dad was a policeman and worked together with his police dog. As such he had to work shifts, and this meant he was at home quite a lot during the day. Mum and Dad could take care of both me and my brother together.

I know that it is easy to see one's childhood in a rosy glow, but nevertheless I must say I am very happy with my childhood.

It was great to grow up in the country, near the forest and the lake. In the summer, Olle and I built huts in the forest, picked blueberries and raspberries, rowed out on the lake in our small rowboat and fished. I remember when I caught my first perch. We grilled it later that evening, and for the first time in my life I thought that perch tasted good!

We were often down by the lake, and when we were not fishing we were bathing, floating on an air-filled rubber mattress, or swimming across to the other side of the lake by trying to race each other. Some summers, Mum and Dad put up a tent in which I loved to both sleep and wake. It was so lovely to wake up when everything was bright orange from the sun that shone through the tent canvas.

In the winter, I sometimes tried to go skating. It didn't go brilliantly, so I was quite happy that Mum had tied a cushion to my bottom.

Apart from these things there was quite a lot to do at home, and Mum always tried to make sure that we children had something to occupy ourselves with. Besides being a policeman, my father was a farmer in his spare time. His big interest was horses. First we had riding horses and then trotting horses, and these horses took up a great deal of his time.

The farm was in great need of repair when we moved in, so there was always something that needed doing. I was often with Dad when he was working at home. Even though I wasn't a particularly great help to him, I watched him work and we talked. When the grownups laid the floor in the basement I was there with them bringing nails and holding planks. When they brought in the hay I rode on the load of hay in the vehicle. Often when Dad was training his trotting horses on the forest roads, he let me ride with him. I felt really close to my dad.

Because we were a bit isolated living out in the country, we did not have many playmates of the same age nearby. Olle and I played much by ourselves, and most of the time we were good friends. However, like most siblings we did tease each other sometimes. Occasionally Olle tried to exploit the situation a bit by, for example, snatching away the chair just when I was about to sit down, or giving me a push when I was on my way down the stairs. But he didn't do such things very often. I was usually stronger than he, and he knew that I might use other "talents" when need be—such as throwing sand in his eyes when we played in the sandpit. He still remembers my "dangerous right foot"!

Yes, I was given a good start in life, but this was not so much because of country air and enjoyable games. Mostly it was because of my parents.

Naturally it is a great burden to have a handicapped child to care for. This is a challenge which might feel overwhelming to some. However, from the beginning my parents had decided to treat me, as far as possible, as an ordinary child. They looked upon me as their daughter Lena who happened to have a handicap — not as a handicapped daughter. It was noticeable that they loved me as the person I was, not for what I could accomplish or what I could not accomplish. This gave me great security.

I was encouraged, like my brother, to devote myself to things in which I was interested. The result was that basically I was never angry or bitter over my situation, for I did not think of my handicap as something negative. I always thought that I was like everyone else. I just did things in a different way.

My parents gave me plenty of time to find out for

myself how to manage different things, instead of attending to me every time I asked for help. This made me stubborn, and usually I wanted to figure out how to master my environment. If, however, I failed, or did not have any more strength, they were always on hand. They did not prevent me from discovering the feeling of disappointment when there was something I could not do. In this way, I had a great opportunity to succeed, but also to cope with failure. I felt such security in knowing that Mum and Dad were always near.

Since my balance was so poor, it often happened that I fell over. One summer's day, our family was invited to visit some friends. Mum and Dad were sitting in the garden talking with our hosts, and Olle and I were playing with their children on the lawn outside. Suddenly I fell and cried out for Mummy. I wanted her to come and lift me up. But my mum didn't want to do this.

"If you crawl over to the fence over there and lean against it you can probably get up." And this I did.

My mum was particularly keen on my being enabled to help myself, for in her work as a physiotherapist she had seen quite a few examples of how terrible it can go when parents overprotect their children.

During my first few years I regularly attended a rehabilitation center for children in Jönköping where I had the opportunity to meet children who had handicaps that were different from mine. I did not feel at home there at all but just thought it was boring. According to my way of looking at things, there was much too little to do. It didn't make it better either that all the children were to have a nap in the afternoon.

Mum let me go with her to the "Children's Hour" at church instead. I felt it was much better to meet children without handicaps and much more fun to play with toys and games, or sing and play instruments.

Mum and Dad encouraged me in a way that made it fun for me to learn new things. For instance, I loved to sit and watch Mum when she did craft work. It didn't take long before I was trying to do the same things she was doing—although I did them with my feet instead. I very much liked to sew, and I could sit for several hours at a time to figure out how to do it. I knew so well how Mum did it, but now it was a matter of adapting so that I could use my feet. I am actually quite proud of the picture with its hens and chickens that I made when I was five years old, and of the tablecloth with mini cross-stitch which I made for my physiotherapist a couple of years later.

At an early age I liked drawing and coloring, and if nobody disturbed me I could go on for several hours. I held my pencil between the big toe and the index toe on my right foot (I'm right-handed, or "right-footed" should I say) and held the paper still with my left foot. This is still the way I do it.

It was good not only for me, but also for Olle, that my parents tried to treat me as a normal child. Because other people did not always have exactly the same attitude as my parents, I was sometimes given special treatment because of my handicap. Kind "aunties" and "uncles" handed my parents little presents in time for my birthday. I did receive these presents, of course, but Mum and Dad always saw to it that there were just as many parcels and presents for Olle when his birthday came around.

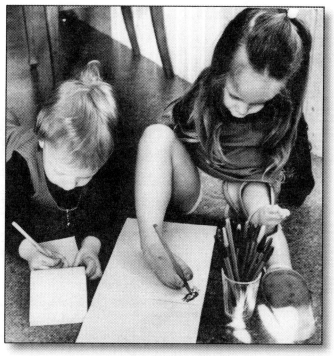

I like to draw and paint. And I was good at it, too!

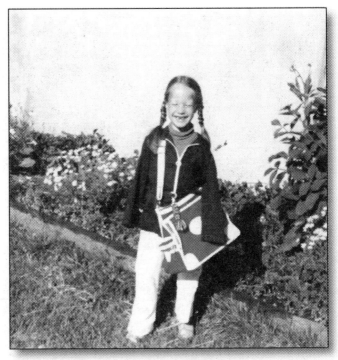

The first day of third grade

4

Prostheses
and a
Priceless Stick

It worked quite well to walk with a prosthesis.

Approximately two or three times a year I had to travel to Uppsala to attend the orthopedic clinic in order to check my prosthetic leg. Approximately once a year—depending on how much I grew—I had to try out a new prosthetic leg.

It was quite a distance from Bankeryd to Uppsala, but it was the orthopedic clinic in Uppsala that specialized in my particular handicap. Even though the journey took several hours I always felt these were cozy family outings, but on the few occasions when I needed a new prosthetic limb it was less cozy. First they wrapped me in wet and warm plaster of Paris around the whole of my left leg and all the way up to my tummy. On the front side of my leg, nearest to my skin, they placed a metal splint. As soon as the plaster had begun to stiffen, they used a sharp knife with which they cut the front side of the plaster. In this way, they created a mold which they could then use to make a new prosthetic limb which fitted me perfectly. It was exciting when they did it, but at the same time it felt a little nauseating.

I became more and more skilled at walking with the help of my prosthetic limb, and my balance became better and better. When I was at home I preferred to jump about on one leg, for everything went a lot smoother then. I even learned to jump up or down the stairs in our home by taking two steps at a time and was duly given the nickname "Little Hoppy." But when I was not at home, the prosthetic limb was invaluable.

When I was ten or eleven years old a big hospital was built in a town nearer to where we lived: Kärnsjukhuset in Skövde, which had its own orthopedic clinic. Since our house was situated in the province of Västergötland

and we also belonged to the correct county council, I no longer needed to make the long journeys to Uppsala in order to lengthen or change my prosthetic limb.

This could have worked fine, but it soon became clear that my prosthetic limbs from Skövde did not work as well as the ones I had before. My weight was not correctly distributed, and so I got blisters which made it difficult to walk. I went there several times with my parents and tried to get them to remake the prosthetic limb so that it would feel more comfortable, but we never felt they really listened to my suggestions or requests. It never worked very well.

One day I was out in the woods together with some other people. Suddenly, something cracked in my left hip. It hurt terribly, and the pain was not like anything I had ever felt before. I was no longer able to walk and had to remove the prosthetic limb. Fortunately, my dad was with me. He carried me the two kilometers (a mile and a quarter) to our home.

Perhaps we should have gone to the hospital, but both my parents and I had lost faith in the hospital in

Skövde. I absolutely refused to go there, and my parents understood me very well.

The pain, however, was terrible. I sat immobile for three days and three nights in a sitting cart, for I could get neither into nor out of bed without increasing the pain. It was not until the fourth night that I was able to slowly move over to my bed, but every time I moved my left leg shook violently and caused me unbearable pain. The only part of my body which I could move was my head, and the only thing I did during these days was read. The Bible was actually my favorite during this time.

For two years I had to sit in a wheelchair. The pain in my left hip gradually disappeared, but I refused to wear the prosthetic limb, for it just caused me more pain. I admit that it was more complicated to be in a wheelchair, but it was also good for me to have a taste of what life in a wheelchair is like. In some circumstances, it could even be an advantage. Because I no longer had to stand on my feet, I could now use them more frequently as hands. When I did my shopping and was about to pay, I no longer had to ask the cashier to take my money out of my pocket. I could easily pick up the money with my feet.

However, there were many other things which I had to learn, whether I was sitting in a wheelchair or not.

The idea for how I could get dressed by myself came during a couple of summer weeks at the rehabilitation home of Bräcke Östergård in Gothenburg.

Several of my handicapped friends had spoken of Bräcke as being a terrible place where they had to go when their parents were to have some relief or a holiday, and I think many of them found it quite hard to cope with being "put away."

For me, however, it was mainly exciting! Because my parents had never made me feel that they needed any relief or holiday without me, when I heard about Bräcke and what one could do there I became very interested. One spring when I accompanied Mum looking at an exhibition of school aids for the handicapped from Bräcke, I met some of their staff and liked them very much. So when summer came, I spent two fine weeks there.

With the help of a physiotherapist, I tried to dress and undress myself. Sweaters were easy. To dress, I just pulled them over my head with the help of my foot. Blouses were no problem either. I buttoned them up first with my feet, and then I pulled them over my head just the way I did with the sweaters. But to put on and take off underpants, slacks and my swimsuit was more difficult because my feet did not reach to my waist. Sometimes I had tried to pull up my slacks by leaning against something which was sticking out, for example the edge of the table, but my garments did not grip well enough. Might a hook do the job?

We tried screwing a hook in the wall, and this worked perfectly. The problem was that I could not carry around a hook which I would have to screw into all toilet walls and dressing-rooms wherever I went. The idea needed to be developed a little, and after some pondering I discovered that the very best solution would be a simple stick with a hook, sufficiently long and handy to be able to hold in my mouth.

No sooner said than done! Such a stick was made for

me, and it worked well from the first moment I tried it. From that day on I have always had my stick with its hook with me wherever I have gone. Occasionally, it has happened that I forgot to bring it, but then I have used whatever is available. Nowadays I know that it works okay with a coat hanger instead. It is much clumsier and it takes much longer to get dressed, but at least it is much better to be able to manage one's toilet visits oneself, without the help of somebody else.

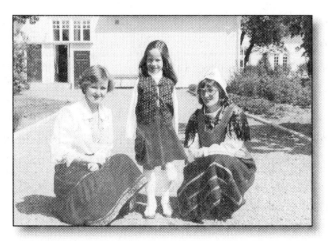

My teacher and helper on the day I finished third grade

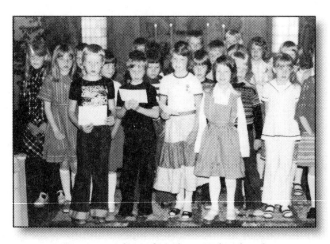

Singing with my friends at Habo church

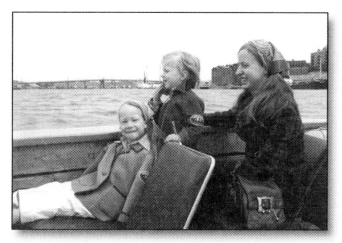

My father took this picture on a family outing.

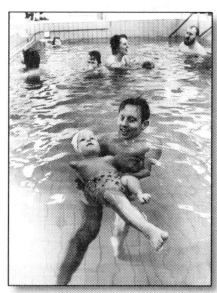

I learned to swim using the Halliwick Method when I was three years old. Here I am with my teacher, Stig Sjölander.

5

School—In My Way

I think Mum and Dad were more nervous than I when the time came for me to start school.

We arrived in good time at the schoolyard. The other children who were also due to start in first-year primary arrived with their parents, and after a while the whole schoolyard was full of people. Most of them were looking at me, of course, and were wondering why I looked the way I did. After a while some of the children had the courage to come forward to have a chat and to ask questions. I feel I answered as well as I could, and when they had got used to my disability it became something natural to them, and I became like any other of their friends.

I had my own specially constructed school table. It was the same height as the chair, and on top of the table there was a shelf where I placed my school books. In this way it was easy for me to get hold of a book with my foot. When the teacher asked a question and we were to put our hands up, I lifted up my leg and waved my foot—if I knew the answer, that is. . . .

I had had a personal assistant already in kindergarten. Pia Lundström was her name, and she remained my assistant until my fifth year. She was a great help to me when it came to doing certain things which I could not manage, but I tried to manage by myself as far as I could. I wanted to because I thought it was fun. Mum and Dad carefully drummed in the message to all adults who had to deal with me, both those at school and those outside school: "Let Lena manage by herself as much as possible. Don't help her unnecessarily."

I liked school, even though naturally there was much that was new and different. If I was unhappy sometimes, it was because I felt that I did not have anyone who was my best friend. In primary school, many girls were walking around with their best friend, but I never had a best friend. I came home to Mum crying sometimes and asking why nobody wanted to be best friends with me. Mum usually explained it by saying that I needed so much help that none of my peers could really cope with it. Instead I had to learn to play with many different children. In this way, it was not always the same people who had to help me with necessary things. Of course, I was sometimes sad even though I understood the reasons, but now I can see that it gave me many friends. Also, I had no problem meeting new people. I became unafraid and did not feel ashamed of my handicap.

The disappointments were sometimes worse for Mum and Dad than they were for me. One term when I was in junior school and using a wheelchair, we were to go on a school journey to Liseberg, the well-known amusement park in Gothenburg. Everybody was looking forward to it. I was, too, but because it was sure to be difficult for me to manage in the wheelchair by myself, Dad came along to lift and carry the wheelchair when necessary. Two of my friends had actually made a firm promise that they would push me in the wheelchair and be with me the whole time. Everything went well for a couple of hours, but suddenly my friends saw something exciting. They ran away and forgot about me completely.

To me it was nothing but a practical problem. I only shouted for Dad and asked him to push me to the place where my classmates had disappeared. But for my dad it was more difficult. Even though he knew that my friends had only been thoughtless and had not intended any harm, it was hard for him to see me left alone in that helpless state.

I suppose it also happened that classmates teased me for my handicap — half in jest and half seriously — but because I never appeared to be upset there was hardly anyone who enjoyed continuing to tease me. "Pegleg" was one nickname I was given in lower-secondary school, and "Loony Macaroony" was another in upper-secondary school, but I just thought they were funny. I was never upset, so potential bullies never had a real chance. As I have said before, Mum and Dad had never tried to hide either my handicap or me. So I was used to people looking and asking. And I had learned early in life that my worth was intrinsic and not in my looks. There was nothing of which I had to be ashamed!

Instead, I learned to make good use of my handicap. When my class did activities in which I could not participate, I invented ways by which I could be involved. I did not want to spend PE lessons sitting on a seat at the side of the room, but playing basketball and handball, for example, was impossible without arms. It was even against the rules! But then it hit me that I could act as a referee, and so I could run around and still take part in the game.

At other times, it was a relief not to have to do everything. Running around in the forest for several hours of orienteering on sports days was not something that I found particularly attractive. I must admit it was much more pleasant to sit at the winning post and tick off the names of those who had finished.

Certain sports were not my cup of tea, but I was so

much better in swimming that it made up for it. I had attended swimming school since I was a young child and had time to practice more than most. So when I was in the sixth year and we were having a sports day in the swimming pools, my classmate Torbjörn and I were chosen to compete on behalf of our class. It was a red-letter day, I felt, for Torbjörn and I beat the other five classes. In spite of this achievement, my report card said only a "2" out of 5 in PE. I thought that was very unfair!

Otherwise I experienced my school years as a fairly painless time. It was probably my mum and dad who had to take the biggest knocks from authorities, school staff and other responsible people who sometimes believed they knew better than my parents.

For example, during my seventh year, I had started to be very independent. I had learned to get dressed and go to the toilet by myself, so I did not need any assistance either in the toilet or in the changing room when we had PE. The only things I sometimes needed help with was to get a book which had slipped too far into my locker or to button my coat right up when it was extra cold. My assistant, who saw that I was managing well by myself, felt that she had too little to do, so she started to help out in the school office instead. When I had finished the seventh year, Dad phoned the headmaster and explained the situation: I no longer needed an assistant, I could manage most things myself, and I could receive help from a classmate with the little things that I could not do by myself. But imagine! It was completely impossible! The headmaster felt that such a great responsibility (as taking out a book from the locker or helping me with my jacket) could absolutely not be put on the pupils. We had meetings and various discussions about this matter, but the school was adamant. This meant that I had to keep my assistant for my eighth year also, even though I felt that I did not need her. We met about once a week and said "hi" to each other.

The office personnel were probably thankful, though, since they received extra help completely free of charge for a whole year.

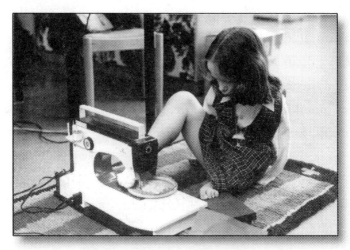

I loved to sew—both by hand and machine—and did this for several hours if I got the chance.

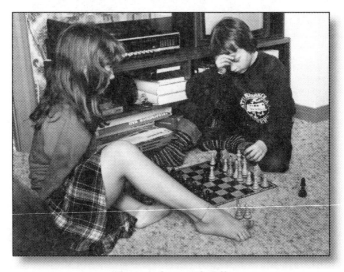

Playing chess with Olle

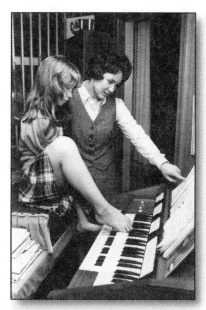

I was interested in music from an early age. Maria Erlandsson taught me to play the organ.

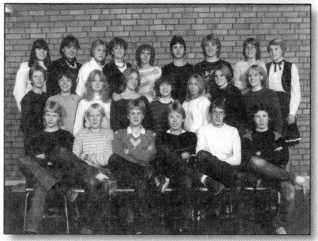

My third year at high school (I'm in the second row, fourth from the right.)

6

"More Secure Is No One Ever"

G od was a natural part of my childhood. It is hard to explain, but in a child's way I just knew that he was there. My parents were — and still are—very active members of a local free church. (A free church is not affiliated with the Catholic or the Protestant State Church.) For them God was as natural as the air they breathed. God meant somebody one could trust, both when things went well and when things went badly, a secure foundation, some-one who loved unconditionally. Naturally, this kind of atmosphere was catching.

It was far from being a severe godliness. They prayed

each evening with Olle and me, and every evening we sang "More Secure Is No One Ever" (all five verses!) together, but there were never any demands that we had to pray this way or that way or behave in a certain way, and yet everything we talked about had God as its center.

Mum and Dad were very much involved with the Habo Covenant Church, one of five (!) churches in our little town and one of the many churches of different denominations in the religious belt which surrounded "Småland's Jerusalem" (the city of Jönköping). Dad had responsibility for the teenagers who were quite often in our home, and Mum was a Sunday School teacher and a Scout leader. Their involvement in the church sometimes took quite a lot of time, but they wanted us to be in on what they were doing. We children never experienced this as the church taking over the family in any way.

We accompanied our parents to church just about every day during the week and also on Sundays. They wanted us to keep quiet during the service, but if occasionally it became boring for us, we could always do some drawings or look in a picture book.

I was a member of the Sunday School, Children's Hour and the children's choir. Later, I joined the Scouts, young people's choir and the teenage group. I watched, listened and pondered it all. Having faith in God gave me a tremendous security, and when I was twelve or thirteen years old my faith became even more firm. Many people in a free church tell of their special experiences of salvation, or how they were saved or how they had made a decision to follow Christ. I cannot say that I have had such an experience. Faith has always been a natural part of my life.

But the church was also important to me in other ways. It was nice for me as a handicapped person to grow up among people who accepted me as the person I was, and who gave me space. I think that my peers who grew up in Habo Covenant Church had approximately a similar experience. In the church there were many different age groups, but the church leadership felt it important to make sure that we who were young would feel that it was also *our* church. They gave us the confidence to do things in our own way.

When we were in our teens we were a close-knit group of about fifteen young people, most of whom were boys. We stuck together through thick and thin. We often took part in various activities in the church. On Sundays, we went to the church services. Many evenings we spent time together in the church's teenage room, or we might hang out in town, or we might spend time in each others' homes.

Most of us had grown up together, so we felt that we knew each other inside out. To them I was simply Lena, a friend who was just one of the gang and definitely not somebody who needed special treatment of any kind.

Sometimes this acceptance was expressed in unexpected ways.

For instance, when I was upset that I could not go with my friends on their canoeing trip, although I wanted with all my heart to go, there was hardly anyone who felt they had reason to feel sorry for me. "Can't you understand that you can't come with us!" they almost indignantly exclaimed.

When I had my eighteenth birthday, according to my friends it was time for me to get my driver's license.

"Why doesn't she take driving lessons?" they wondered among themselves—and they didn't mean anything bad.

But for me to get a driver's license was, of course, not as easy as for them. I had applied for a grant which would enable me to have a car adapted to my special needs, but it wasn't until this had been done that I could start to take driving lessons. Then it wasn't so long until I passed the test.

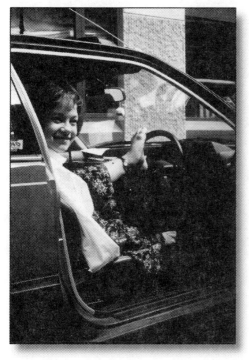

Practicing my driving

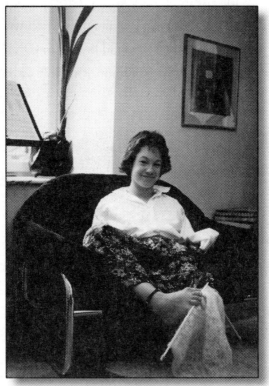

Knitting in my living room

7

Like a
Fish in
the Water

The Swedish national anthem was ringing out from the loudspeakers at the World Championships in Gothenburg — for my sake. It was lovely warm weather, and the sun was shining from a sky which was almost completely cloudless. Around my neck hung the gold medal, and it was a wonderful feeling to have earned it. I had just won the fifty-meter backstroke event.

I felt it had been so easy. Many of my friends had been practicing so hard for several years in order to stand where I was standing now. I found it hard to grasp that I was now a member of the national team.

Who would have thought this when I was three years old and started to accompany Mum, Dad and Olle to the swimming pools in Jönköping? It was then that I started to swim according to the so-called Halliwick method. This method came from England, and the main thing about it was that it maintained that children could learn to swim without the use of floating aids.

Parents and swimming instructors were with us children in the swimming pool all the time. They taught us not to be afraid of the water. Stig Sjölander, a pastor in Jönköping who also had a disabled child of his own, had heard of the Halliwick method. He started a course for all children with a handicap who wanted to learn to swim. It is a well-known fact that moving about in water is good exercise for the whole body, and for a disabled person it is a fine way of training muscles that would otherwise not get much exercise.

We went as a family, except on the occasions when my dad was working. Swimming was something that we all felt was great fun. We met once a week. To start with we played "Follow John," "The Kettle Is Boiling" and other water games. Each participant had one or two parents with them, and sometimes brothers and sisters as well, so the swimming pool was usually crowded.

When some of us had become a little more used to water we tried to float on the arms of one of our parents. I was five years old when Mum and Dad could let go of me and I dared to float by myself. A year later I had received more training and was able to swim. Because I had learned to float on my back, it was most natural for me to start with the backstroke.

To start with I just kicked with my legs and worked up speed while kicking, but soon I was confident enough to turn over onto my tummy and start breaststroke. Then it was only my head that stuck up out of the water! I loved to swim under the water, but sometimes I floated much too easily. Other people at the swimming pool joked with me saying that I floated like a cork whereas my dad sank like a stone. . . .

When I was in the second year at school and accompanied my classmates to swimming classes, I already knew how to swim. I was allowed to jump straight into the big pool, complete two hundred meters swimming, and I received a little badge to prove my accomplishment.

Later, when I progressed to learning different swimming techniques, the butterfly stroke came to suit me best. It became my special event. In this event, one lets one's body move in an undulating movement while working with one's legs and feet to get up speed. One tries to imitate a dolphin's way of swimming. I tried to use this technique also when I did the backstroke.

Now I was standing there with my gold medal at a world championship. Three years previously I had not thought that I would ever start to swim again.

I had actually been practicing diving from the diving board for three school terms. We had been diving from a board which was one meter high, and I had enjoyed it. But during the fourth term, when everybody was to start diving from the three-meter board, I was advised not to continue, because it was not considered good for my head since I had no hands with which to part the water. This led me to conclude that this was the end of all my swimming.

But I continued with other sports. The Swedish Covenant Church arranged volleyball practice every Wednesday evening and Saturday morning. The practice was in a sports hall in Habo. I got quite a hard introduction to this game. During the first practice I headed the ball for half an hour without any break at all, and the following day I had a terrible headache. This first practice, however, made me fearless when the ball came towards me, and it didn't hurt when I headed the ball either.

Our team sometimes went to play volleyball against other teams. Such games were arranged by various churches in our district. We enjoyed playing, even though our girls' team was soon knocked out, but after this we could enjoy watching the big boys from Tibro playing.

Then, in 1983, someone called me from Jönköping. They were going to start a sports club for disabled people and were wondering if I wanted to join in the swimming. I had already been featured in various newspapers, so a number of people knew about me. They reasoned that perhaps other disabled people would be encouraged to start to swim if they knew I practiced there. No sooner said than done. Having stopped training for almost two years, I now started again.

I participated in a race here and there. Among other places I took part in a race in Finland and enjoyed it. When our swimming club was invited to participate in the Swedish Championships for the disabled in 1986, people were nudging me, wondering if I wanted to go.

The competition took place in Stockholm, and I was to swim in four different events for the disabled: the twenty-five-meter butterfly stroke, twenty-five-meter backstroke, twenty-five-meter breaststroke, and twenty-five-meter freestyle. There were many lanes and many different times of which to keep track, particularly because disabled sports at that time were divided into a multitude of different classes, much more so than today. Just keeping track of which lane and which time was almost like a competition in itself!

But it went well. I came in second in both backstroke and freestyle, and I took home two silver medals. I came in last in breaststroke in my class, but I made up for it in the butterfly stroke, for I won, and at the same time I broke the Swedish record.

I was as surprised as everybody else! The provincial team leaders got their eyes opened, and before the Swedish championships were over I had qualified for a place in the Swedish national team for the disabled.

Oh, dear! Now I suddenly had to take my swimming seriously. I had to practice four times a week instead of once. Now and then I had to take part in a training camp for the national team. Jan-Åke Sundbring, more well-known as Knasen, was the trainer at the swimming pools in Råslätt where I practiced. He had previously been a trainer for top swimmers, but had quit. Now he took me under his wing and became my personal trainer for a number of years to come.

When training most intensively, I swam between two thousand and three thousand meters every session. Sometimes I swam alone, sometimes with other disabled swimmers, and sometimes with the top swimmers from Jönköping's swimming club. Some people may well have thought I lived in the swimming pool! It was important to make my normal leg stronger— as strong as possible — and at the same time "find the dolphin movement in my body." This meant causing the movements of my right leg to work like a rhythmic wave from the toes, and up to my head and back again. This was the most special and effective feature. I made good use of my musical ability and my feeling for rhythm, even in the water.

Knasen and I became good friends. He appreciated my will to practice and also my energy. I, on the other hand, appreciated the fact that he had a goal and knew where he was going, and I also appreciated the way he was quite demanding. He set goals for me, then broke them down into smaller goals. He made me train towards these all the time, and this spurred me on.

In spite of the fact that I was chosen to represent Sweden in the World Championships, this was nevertheless a disappointment to me. I had been having many exciting dreams about the countries where the World Championships were likely to be held, but then it was announced that the chosen place was Gothenburg. One and a half hour's journey from home! That was not exactly where I would have liked to go.

And now I was standing here anyway, on the World Championship pedestal in Gothenburg, with the sun shining in my eyes and the Swedish national anthem resounding in my ears. I tried to really think about how it felt to be best in the world. The feeling was not quite as strong as I had imagined, but, of course, it was a great feeling anyway to be the winner.

Before the World Championships were over, I had taken yet another gold medal and one bronze medal.

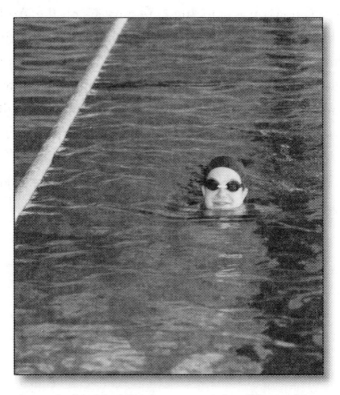

As a swimmer, I had the chance to travel to different places.

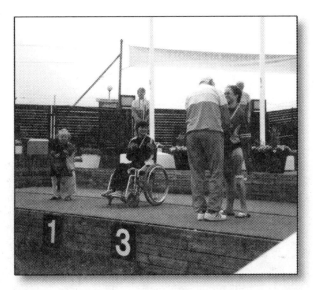

Third prize for the fifty-meter freestyle at the 1986 World Championships in Gothenburg

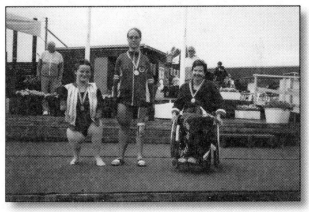

I had to practice swimming in order to become a champion swimmer. My goal was a gold medal at the Paralympic Games in Seoul, South Korea.

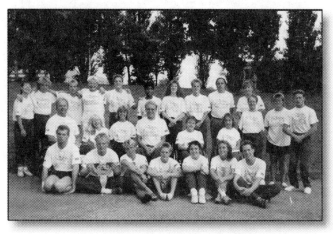

*I was on the Swedish national team in the Paralympics
(middle row, third from right).*

8

Towards the Olympic Games in Seoul

We Swedish swimmers were superior to everyone else during the World Championships in Gothenburg. I think we took forty-two gold medals between us.

These years in the mid-1980s were enormously successful for Swedish disabled swimmers. As a nation, we held our own very well against "big" countries like Germany, Great Britain and the United States, and sometimes we were even better than they were. It was almost effortless.

Naturally, it was far from the truth that it depended only on me! There were five or six Swedish swimmers who were outstanding in their classes (and there were many classes for different types of disabilities), and when they competed in their events— perhaps four or five each — they won many medals. The two successful twins, Magdalena and Gabriella Tjernberg, were among these swimmers, and they became good friends of mine.

The trainers as well as the swimmers were of great importance, especially when it came to finding the funds for training camps and races to which we could otherwise not have been able to afford to go.

This was the case when we were travelling to the Nordic Championships on the Faroe Islands. Bengt Olofsson, the chairman of the Disabled Swimmers' Association, had made an agreement with the Defense Department, which on this occasion allowed us to fly in a Hercules military aircraft to and from the race. We sat in chairs which were like hammocks, with our safety belts fastened and earplugs in. The noise was terrible, but the flight was exciting. The journey home was even more exciting with such bad weather that no other planes were allowed to fly. It was the bumpiest flight I have experienced, but we made it safely home and were happy that we didn't have to wait for the better weather.

By the way, I have an amusing anecdote from the training camp at Tranås. Having been to Linköping for a swimming show we were driving back to Tranås. I had quite recently got my driving license and was driving, with my passengers Annelie Österström and Marie-Louise Freij. We had stopped briefly at a McDonald's (which in itself is just about illegal if one is a member of the national team) when I noticed that I had left the keys in the car. And the car was locked!

We rang the police, and after a while they came to help us, but initially they hesitated to open the car. They looked from me who had no arms to my companions, Annelie and Marie-Louise, who were unusually short, and back to me again and said: "And which of you is the driver of this car, then?" for my car, a Honda Prelude, looked like any ordinary car. The steering wheel is in the normal place (I steer with my right foot); the accelerator and the brake have just been lengthened a little to fit my left foot. The light switch and the indicators are placed in the headrest and are controlled by the movements of my head.

I cannot remember if I had to show the police my driver's license or not, but everything went well. Five police cars came in the end— out of pure curiosity!— to help us, and after some discussion they managed to open the car, and we continued our journey back to the training camp.

In 1987, the year after the World Championships, the European Championships were scheduled to take place in France. I was really in good shape at the time. I took four gold medals in four different events, but if I am to be really honest I can no longer remember my times or what events I won. Well, of course I remember that I beat the world record for the butterfly stroke!

Not only did our national team take part in the European Championships, but we also took part in various other competitions and training camps. Once I met a Frenchman who, like me, had no arms. We were sitting outside one day playing a card game with some friends from the training camp. The Frenchman and I had our own way of holding the cards, of course; we held them with our feet. While enviously studying his card technique, I concluded that it was quite a lot easier if you had long toes—quite different from my toes, which are the size of little cocktail sausages!

But now the time was drawing near to what many of us considered to be the most important goal of our training—the Olympic Games for the handicapped, or the Paralympic Games, which were held in Seoul, South Korea, following the Olympic Games. This was my goal, even though I had moved to Stockholm and started to study at Stockholm's Music Conservatory. The swimming and all the training swallowed up much of my time. I started to ask myself what I was doing. Was it really worth all the hard work? I had never even enjoyed training!

What drove me was not my successes, but rather my desire to travel, and also the camaraderie between us swimmers during the training camps and at the competitions. There was many an evening when I talked

with a roommate on every subject under the sun: anything from a disabled person's situation to our thoughts
about life and about God. I discovered that compared to
many of these friends I was fortunate to have had such
a wonderful childhood and parents who not only loved
me, but who also showed me the way to faith.

From time to time, I was asked to tell them why I had
never felt angry or bitter over my handicap, and sometimes I could perhaps help someone by just listening. It
was very much these conversations that caused me to
feel that it was meaningful to continue with training.

In January 1988, with ten months left until the
Paralympic Games in Seoul, I had nevertheless had
enough. I wanted to quit. I told both God and myself
that "next week I am going to the trainer of the national
team to tell him that I will quit." A couple of days later,
however, I had a phone call from a woman whom I
knew had been praying for me for several years. She told
me that while praying for me she had felt that God
wanted her to phone me to encourage me concerning
the swimming. She did not know about my plans at all,

but the phone call made me change my mind. I went on with the training and became a part of the Swedish Paralympic team.

The opening ceremony of the Paralympic Games was absolutely the greatest experience of all. More than 70,000 spectators crowded the stands when approximately 4,000 disabled athletes from 60 nations marched into the Olympic Stadium. The Swedish team consisted of 132 people. Music was pouring out of the loudspeakers, while giant screens were showing close-ups of all the participants as they came walking in. The Olympic flame was lit. The whole opening ceremony was festive and colorful— almost as festive and colorful as the opening of the ordinary Olympics— and I thought it was such a great feeling to be together with so many celebrating and happy people. I must admit that I was thinking, "It will probably be like this when we get to heaven!"

Also, the whole city of Seoul was affected by the Olympics. In some other cities that have hosted both the Olympics and the Paralympics, the Games have

been more or less over after the first Olympics, the
"ordinary" Olympics. But it wasn't like that in Seoul.
The whole city seemed to think that the Paralympics
were at least as important as the Olympics for the athletes who were not disabled. The Paralympics in Seoul
had its own mascot—a bear. The first banners and
posters were changed for new ones, and there were
flowers and flags everywhere.

They had made one big mistake, though. When the
Olympic village was being built, they had forgotten to
build it in a handicap-friendly way. At the last minute
the organizers had to build a new Olympic village, nine
high-rise buildings with apartments suitable for the disabled, and there we were installed.

The Games were well-attended and well-covered by
the press and television. There were crowds of spectators in the stands, including people from the many different churches in Seoul. They cheered the participants
with various kinds of banners and pennants, and
sometimes they had even learned a supporters' chant
from the country that they had decided to support. It

was really great when everyone was cheering for "their" country.

I was entered for four events: twenty-five-meter back-stroke, butterfly stroke, freestyle, and breaststroke. My best event was the butterfly stroke, and naturally I was banking on this most of all. The evening before this event, however, I was informed that there were not enough countries entered for this particular event, for one country had withdrawn. The twenty-five-meter butterfly stroke event was thus cancelled.

The evening *Aftonbladet's* reporter Leif-Åke Josefsson noticed this and wrote as follows:

> *Lena Maria Johansson is a victim of how the sports for the disabled is turning out today. . . . Lena Maria's case is only one of many during these Paralympic Games which have been marred by chaos and confusion. In her special event there weren't the four obligatory partici-pants. Consequently there was no race! Lena Maria had to be contented with other*

swimming styles, a few fifth places and a few sixth places, but thus no gold medal during this "Gold Rush" Olympics. Will she have the endurance to persevere until the next Olympic Games? In Barcelona, 1992, there will be a new and better chance. . . .

Admittedly I was a bit disappointed, but I hardly felt I was a victim. I felt happy over my fourth place in backstroke, fifth place in freestyle and sixth place in breaststroke. I was terribly tired of training and instead wanted to devote myself to singing and music.

I never did try to get to Barcelona. The Paralympic Games in Seoul was my last competition, for it is just as the wise saying goes, "One should stop when things are at their best."

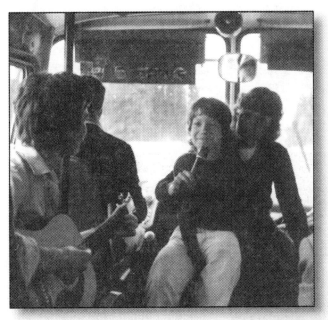

*Leading the singing on the
way to a church outing*

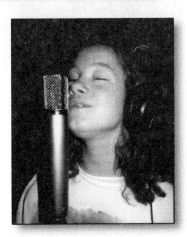

I really gave myself to music.

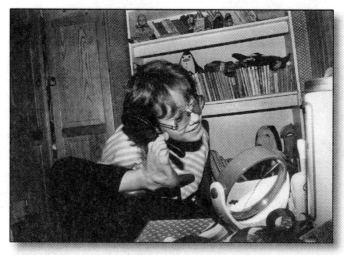

Getting ready

9

With Singing
and
Synthesizer

I don't think there was anyone who really believed in my voice to start with, but this did not particularly worry me.

Singing and music were a natural part of my life from my very first years. Musically I was brought up on a diet of Christian hymns and Dad's recordings of The Oak Ridge Boys. Both Mum and Dad and many of our relatives liked to sing and play instruments, so I couldn't help but try, too!

Sometimes while I was still a little girl I was asked to sing at family gatherings. They put me to stand on a chair so that everyone could see me. We had family reunions several times a year, and on Christmas Day there was a special tradition. We went to a retirement home to sing some of our finest Christmas carols for the elderly people. I remember it as being very enjoyable.

Added to this, the church, and also the local music school, helped to increase my interest. In many free churches, music is a central part of church life, and the Covenant churches in Habo and Bankeryd were no exception. I started by singing in the children's choir in Bankeryd's Covenant Church. That was also the time when I composed my first song. "I Want to Be a Friend" was the name of the little tune. My dad wrote the text to go with it, and we used it frequently in the children's choir.

Because I could keep a tune at a tender age, I was sometimes asked to sing solos. I didn't mind this at all. Quite the opposite! I enjoyed standing in the middle of a group of people and being the center of attention. This was good training for what was to happen later in my life. I started so early that I have never felt nervous about singing before many people.

The electric organ became my instrument in the local music school. This was practical because we had an electric organ, so I could take my music lessons at home. From my third school year onwards, a teacher, Maria Erlandsson, came to our home once a week to teach me. She used to be the conductor of the children's choir at church. She let me sit on a stool somewhat higher than the organ in order to allow my feet to be high enough.

When I was in lower-secondary school and wanted to continue taking lessons to play the church organ, the school authorized somebody to make me a set of two special stools as a support for the regular music stool, so that my feet would be able to reach the keys from the right height. Naturally it was impossible for me to use the foot pedals, too, but I enjoyed learning to play the great old hymns anyway.

In my ninth year, I started to take music lessons at the community music school in Jönköping. I was not particularly good at singing, and there was, as I said before, just about nobody who believed in my voice. But I thought music was great!

The time came when I was to choose which track in upper-secondary school I wanted to follow. I was thinking back and forth: My report cards were not brilliant — I was about average perhaps — and I was not actually interested in choosing subjects where I would have to spend a lot of time studying, even if (against all expectations) I would be accepted there. My dream was to train to become a secretary or an office worker, but when I heard that there was a two-year social track combined with music, I became very interested.

However, there was just this one problem: There were many more than I who wanted to be accepted there! My marks were not good enough. Not by a long shot!

And yet, against all odds, I was accepted. It was my good fortune that I was offered one of the extra places after having shown my musical talents at an entrance test. I think it was mainly because I was disabled that I was accepted, for I wasn't exactly a star in either singing or instrumental music at that time.

As a student in the Per Brahe School's music track, I

found the studies enormously stimulating and enjoyed my two years there very much indeed. They were my two best school years without a doubt! We took our music subjects in a specially built music building, where we spent the greater part of every twenty-four hours. Even though the lessons usually started at eight o'clock in the morning, we students used to be in the music building until nine o'clock at night, for that's when the burglar alarm was turned on. Consequently, everybody had to leave then.

One year we put on the musical *West Side Story* for a week, and this was also fabulous. I was in the orchestra and played the synthesizer. We also did a couple of school trips to London where we had the opportunity to see performances of "real" musicals.

At the same time I was also trying to lead the youth choir back home — in the Covenant Church in Habo. After all my years in the children's choir I had now advanced to the youth choir, and I was soon asked if I wished to lead it. Naturally, I could not direct it with my non-existent arms, but it is not arms that make a choir sing, but what is learned at the practices. So when the choir performed I just stood in front of them and led by my own singing and showing with my head, mouth and eyes what they were supposed to do.

The choir became quite good, and we were asked by other churches if we would go and hold concerts. Through these contacts I also started to perform by myself and hold my own concerts in churches in the provinces of Västergötland and Småland.

The two years went quickly, but I had the opportunity to do a third year in the music school. I so very much wanted to occupy myself with music in the future, but what was I to do when my time at the school was over? Many of my school friends were thinking of applying to different music colleges. This is what I also decided to do.

I was planning to apply to Stockholm's Music Conservatory, but before I did this my music teacher, Lasse Persson, and I went up to Stockholm to meet the head of the individual musicians' course to which I wished to apply. I needed to get to know some things about the course, but the Music Conservatory also needed to get to know some things about me. We talked through the various parts of the course and how these might work out for me if I went. The school leadership saw no problem with my being disabled and encouraged me to apply.

During the entrance tests each one of us had fifteen minutes to show our musical ability. Of the different things I did during this test the one I can remember best was the marvelously funny song I sang called "I Am So Ugly" while accompanying myself on the synthesizer. Soon afterwards I received the news that I had been accepted as one of the four students for the individual musicians' course. I am sure that "I Am So Ugly" played a part in this!

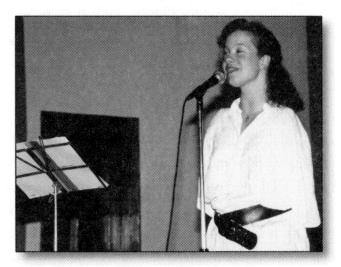

Singing at a concert

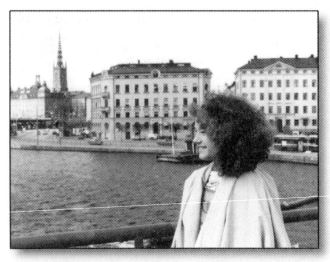

*This picture was taken in Stockholm when
I was a student at the music conservatory.*

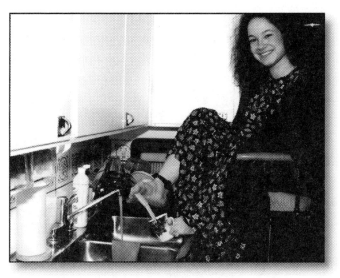

Doing my own washing up

10

Not "Lena Johansson" — The One Without Arms

Lena Johansson, Lena Johansson, Lena Johansson, Lena Johansson, Lena Johansson.

I did not need to look in the telephone directory to know that there were lots of people in Stockholm with the same name as me.

I had no desire at all to become "the Lena Johansson without arms," so I had to think of something before I moved to Stockholm. In the province of Hälsingland I had three second cousins who all had double names, which I felt sounded very nice. Since I had two names, both Lena and Maria, I decided to start using both names as my first name; so, from the autumn term when I moved to Stockholm, people came to know me as Lena Maria.

Moving from home to a completely new town full of strangers is probably not easy for anybody. I thought it was exciting and fun, but at the same time I found it a bit difficult. We were three classmates from Jönköping who had been accepted at the Music Conservatory, and we were each allotted a room on the same floor in a street called Tegnérgatan. It was a relief not to have to move up to Stockholm completely by myself, but even better to be neighbors with my two friends.

Now it was time for me to manage completely on my own for the very first time. At home, I had always had Mum to help me with just about everything, but now I had to be able to manage cleaning, washing and ironing, cooking, washing up and everything else one does in a household. I didn't know if I would manage it, so for the first six months I had a house helper who came once a week in order to do mainly the cleaning and ironing. In a way, this was a splendid arrangement, but when it transpired that approximately every three weeks a new house helper came whom I had to train, I got tired of it. I found it was easier to do it all myself and be independent of the house helper's hours. It went well, even though there were times when I found that it was inconvenient because it took up so much time.

From the beginning, I enjoyed studying at the Music Conservatory. The Faculty for Individual Musicians where I was studying gave me great freedom in shaping the schedule myself. They even allowed me to choose which singing teacher I wanted. I chose the singer Lena Ericsson, who sometimes accepted students and who was even a member of the school's selection committee.

We met regularly, usually in her home, and I had time to learn an enormous amount during the four years she was my teacher. From the very beginning she told me that she did not intend to take special notice of my disability. "It is up to you to tell me what you can, or cannot, do," she said, and this suited me perfectly.

She made a great effort to make me really use my body when I sang, to make me sing with all I have got, and to dare sing out and communicate what I wanted to communicate. "A voice is a feeling," she said.

To start with she probably felt I was a little reserved, but I tried to absorb as much as possible of what she told me, for I really did want to develop my voice so that it could touch other people. I wanted to communicate my faith through my singing, and one way I could do this was by continuing to hold concerts in different churches. I had met a pianist, Hans-Inge Magnusson, with whom I started to perform in various parts of Sweden.

Naturally, I also wanted to communicate my faith at the Music Conservatory. I often met with Hans-Inge and a few other student friends to exchange thoughts about the meaning of life, and about God. It was always stimulating and interesting, but I who had been brought up in the area near "Småland's Jerusalem" (Jönköping) soon came to realize that I had never thought through why I believed in God or why I felt and thought the way I did about other things, too. Now when I was forced to argue the reasons for my opinions, I noticed that I had taken over quite a number of thought patterns and ideals from my parents without any deep reflection. I did not have a real foundation of my own to stand on.

Afterwards, I think it was a useful and necessary experience, but at the time it was frustrating. I questioned, I pondered, I prayed to God, and I read the Bible.

Gradually, my faith could stand on its own two legs, and this made it much stronger. I also experienced that God was near me and frequently helping me by doing little miracles in my everyday life. I know that some people would probably reason that there might have been other explanations for many of these miracles, but to me they were meaningful signs of God's care and that he was near to me. This caused me to feel even more sure that I wanted to sing in order to point others to him.

This is why it felt altogether right when Lena Ericsson asked me if I wanted to go along and sing a song at the Gröna Lund entertainment park in Stockholm. She was to perform there one evening and wanted me to contribute a song. I felt this would be great fun and chose to sing one of Duke Ellington's wonderful songs, "Heaven."

It was a warm spring evening. It had just become dark, but Gröna Lund was lit up by lamps and spotlights. It was terribly crowded—perhaps because entrance was free on this particular evening—but this did not make me nervous. I sang my little song, but on my way out I was stopped by Magnus Härenstam, the master of ceremonies, who ushered me back to the stage again! There was Bosse Parnevik, the famous Swedish imitator.

I soon came to understand the reason behind it all. I had been chosen by "Sällskapet Stallbröderna," an association for people who are in entertainment, to receive their Bosse Parnevik scholarship. I was given flowers and a check for ten thousand Swedish kronor to enable me to continue studying music. Lena Ericsson knew about the scholarship, of course. Her suggestion that I should sing had only been a pretext to get me there without my having to know anything beforehand. And I could never have imagined this! It was a great surprise and an enormous encouragement.

The evening papers also took note of the scholarship.

One thing led to another. The *Aftonbladet* carried an article in which they wrote about my life in Stockholm, about my swimming, and about gearing up for the Paralympic Games, and at the same time they splashed a very large picture in the centerfold of me sitting in my car with my foot on the steering wheel.

This in turn led two TV workers in Umeå, Henrik Burman and Sven-Erik Frick, to become interested in me. They were just in the process of planning a few documentary programs, and when they read about me they phoned and wanted me to join them to tell them about my life in Stockholm. I said "yes" straight away, for it sounded incredibly enjoyable.

By this time, I had actually moved to an apartment of my own. At the time of my arrival in Stockholm I had applied properly for an apartment and joined the long line of applicants, but I had also asked that my application be allowed to jump the line, as disabled people are allowed to do. Some people had told me that it would be impossible to jump the line in Stockholm unless I was registered there, and others said that it was impossible to obtain an apartment in the center of the city.

However, just before Christmas, before my first term was even finished, I was informed that I had been allowed to jump the line, and soon afterwards came an offer of an apartment. It consisted of one-and-a-half rooms with a kitchen in an old but newly renovated house on Kungsholmen—with a supermarket and an underground station in the same block, and only a five-minute walk from the Central Station.

Was this fate, good fortune—or God? It was perfect for me anyway.

The flat had not been specially adapted to the needs of disabled people, but I didn't think I needed this anyway. If a person has other obstacles to movement this is sometimes necessary, but I preferred to have an ordinary apartment. I wanted—and I still want—to adapt myself to other people's needs as much as possible, rather than the other way around. In the kitchen I just needed a stool on wheels. It was a little higher than the sink to enable me to do the cooking and washing up.

It was in this apartment that Sven-Erik and Henrik

met me for the first time. I treated them to a sponge cake I had baked myself (which I later understood had impressed them a lot) and we made a good contact.

During the next few weeks they followed me around wherever I went and whatever I did, whether it was training for the Paralympic Games, practicing singing and playing at the Music Conservatory, making tea, going to see my parents, going for a drive in my car, buying milk or cooking food. I noticed that they were used to making people feel relaxed in front of the camera, so all the time the filming went very well.

It was more difficult to talk about myself and my opinions of my life as a handicapped person. Nowadays I am used to speaking in public about most things that concern my life, but then it was almost the first time, and it was difficult for me to express myself.

In spite of this, the program turned out very well. I thought so, and so, too, apparently did many other people who turned on their televisions to watch *Goal in Sight* when it was aired one evening during the autumn of 1988. Many people contacted me—through letters and in other ways—and it still happens that people come up to me to talk about this TV program.

It was even thought to be so good that it was selected to represent Sweden in a Christian TV festival, the so-called Kristoval, in Holland, the following year. *Goal in Sight* won the hearts of both the jury and the public and was voted the best. The reasons went like this:

> *This is the portrait, full of life and good humor, of a young disabled woman who has decided to live an independent life. Through their ability to treat this fantastic woman as an equal, the producers have avoided condescension, excesses and emotionalism. They communicate a message of hope to the disabled and their relatives, while stating the many physical, psychological, social and economic problems that Lena Maria meets in her daily life. This document of hope and faith deserves to be spread widely.*

Many countries wanted to buy the film. I had become Lena Maria to more people than I could ever have imagined. The snowball had started to roll.

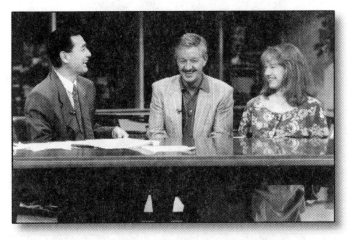

I never imagined that the TV program in Japan would be so successful. Here I am being interviewed by Mr. Kume, presenter of News Station.

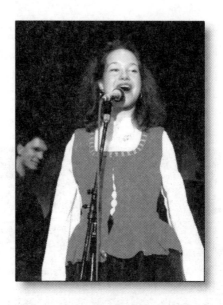

I really enjoy singing at concerts.

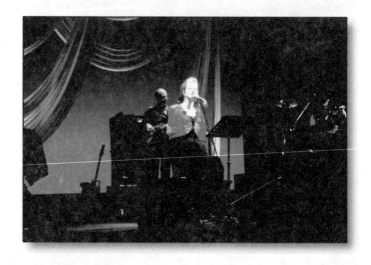

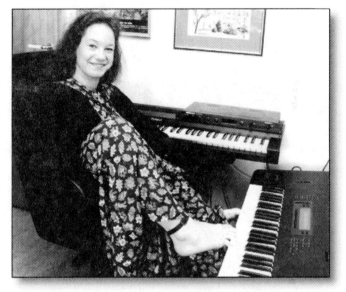

Practicing is fun.

11

With the Goal in Sight— But Why?

G oal in Sight came to mean much more than I could have imagined. Since my birth, my mum had had a strong assurance that something special was going to happen to me during my twenties. Looking back now I believe it was the TV program, for it led to incredibly many things during the next few years.

I had many reactions from viewers. There were those who just wrote to tell me how admirable they felt I was and so on, but the letters where people told me of how they had been encouraged and helped by the program made me even happier.

The publicity caused me to receive even more inquiries about concerts. To tell people about Jesus through my singing was something that I really wanted to do, so naturally I enjoyed receiving more and more opportunities to sing.

During this spring term I had so many engagements that my pianist, Hans-Inge, did not always have the time to come along. Sara Fält, a friend from upper-secondary school, sometimes took his place as accompanist, but soon I started to work with another pianist, Anders Wihk, on a regular basis. I had met him when I had been conducting temporarily a youth choir in Stockholm. At the time, he had recently returned from the United States after completing five years of studies at Berkeley College of Music. Anders did not perhaps completely share my taste in music, but he shared my longing to use music to glorify God.

And then I had an audience with Queen Silvia of Sweden! During the spring of 1989 the queen was about to visit a congress about the disabled in the United States. One of the reasons for her going there was to launch a book about sports for the disabled for which she herself had taken the initiative and to which she had also written the foreword. Some people at the court had seen Burman and Frick's film about me and wanted to take it with them to show at the congress. They felt that I was a good example of a disabled athlete, and so an abridged version of the film was made.

When the queen came home from the United States she wanted to meet me, and so I was given an audience. I felt it was a real honor to meet her so privately, even though naturally I was not completely alone with her. The two filmmakers, Henrik Burman and Sven-Erik Frick, were there, and also Gert Engström, who had been to the United States with the queen, and a lady-in-waiting. We had been given half an hour to talk with the queen, but it was so pleasant that we continued a bit longer.

Queen Silvia asked much about my life and what dreams and hopes I had for the future. Soon the audience was over, and after some newspaper reporters took photographs of us, we said good-bye. The queen left, somewhat delayed, for her next engagement.

When we came out into the courtyard we noticed that it had been raining. I had only taken a few steps towards my car when I slipped and fell head over heels. It happens from time to time that I fall over, and mostly it goes well, but this time everything was spinning when I tried to get up.

Gert Engström was worried and wanted to call for an ambulance immediately, but I felt this was completely unnecessary. After a while I had to give in, though, for I quite simply could not get up, and my left foot had started to hurt very much.

The prosthetic limb had come halfway off at my fall, and at the same time my foot had been wrenched around— that was why it hurt so much. The ambulance came, and they took me to the hospital at lightning speed. Even though my foot was still hurting, I felt it was a great experience to ride in an ambulance in Stockholm! It went fast because all the other cars gave way to us the whole time.

After arriving at the hospital I had to sit and wait by

myself for a good long while, but this did not matter to me. I sat and sang a little to myself and talked to God and asked him to help me. I was booked for a concert the following weekend and did not want to cancel it, so I said, "Now, God, you'll have to see to it that I'll be well enough to be able to go."

After waiting for three hours I was allowed to see a doctor, was examined and X-rayed. On the films they could see three cracks in my left foot, so it was no wonder that it was hurting. The doctor gave me some pills for the pain, and then a friend drove me home. I took one of the pills and went to bed.

When I woke the next morning, I discovered to my surprise that all the pain had disappeared. Naturally it still hurt when I tried to move my foot, but the constant pain was gone, and this made me exuberant.

This is good, God! Please continue like this! I thought and went to a center where they have aids for the disabled. It was impossible to jump on one leg all the time, so I was glad when they loaned me a wheelchair. But I was even happier when I came home and found twenty yellow tulips hanging on my door. They were from the queen with her "Get Well" greetings. It is not every day one gets flowers from Queen Silvia. . . .

But a few days later, I was to have a singing lesson at my teacher, Lena Ericsson's apartment, and this was a little problematic. Her apartment was situated on the third floor, and there was no elevator. I knew that I could not jump up all the flights of stairs, for then I would not have the strength to sing afterwards. But perhaps the swelling had gone down enough for me to support myself somewhat on it? I tried gingerly to walk with my prosthetic limb. To my great surprise it worked. And after I had coped with the singing lesson I decided that it should be possible to go ahead with the concert also. And it was!

A few weeks later, I received a phone call from Gert Engström who told me that Queen Silvia wanted to give me a scholarship from the king and queen's wedding fund in order that I should be able to continue studying music. I was given ten thousand Swedish crowns, which I used for my journey to the United States to study "black gospel" at a big gospel convention there.

Being a voice in this gigantic choir of twenty-five hundred people (of whom only five were Caucasian), with its several conductors, was a fantastic experience. The big, solid ladies all around me sang so that the ground rocked. That's where I learned what real gospel singing is!

Back in Sweden I worked on my scales and singing lessons, and at the same time Anders and I had a number of concerts. It was all go all the time.

During the spring of 1991, even more happened when a short version of *Goal in Sight* was aired in Japan. It was during prime-time on the popular program *News Station* on TV Asahi, which is one of the biggest TV channels in Japan.

There were many reactions from the Japanese viewers. Perhaps the main reason for this was that they have a completely different attitude toward the disabled. For the most part, they look upon disabled people as second-class citizens. Through this TV program they received a completely different picture.

The producer, a woman by the name of Kaori Asamoto, decided to send a Japanese team to Sweden to make their own program about me. Their film team was with me in Stockholm for one week, and they had time to go with me to a great number of places. They were with me at one of my concerts, but they also filmed me at home to show how I coped with my everyday life.

The program was aired one Friday evening, and there were many Japanese viewers. The following Friday I was at the *News Station* studio to be interviewed and to sing on their program which was broadcast live. I found all of this very exciting, especially as it indicated that there was a possibility that I could continue with my music even after finishing college.

In the summer of 1991, when I graduated from the Music Conservatory in Stockholm, I was completely sold on the idea of singing for a few years to come, and I was grateful that I would be able to do this full-time. I loved to sing. In the autumn I was back in the United States again. My pianist, Anders, and I had been invited to minister in song in various churches in the United

States for almost two months. Among other places, we were asked to take part in a live broadcast of a service in the Crystal Cathedral in Los Angeles.

The tour was intense. We did fifty-six different performances, of which thirty were whole concerts, within fifty-four days. It just became too much. When we came home I did not feel well. I was at home with my parents over Christmas, but I slept almost the entire time. Physically I was probably in quite good condition, but not mentally. I had lost my desire for everything. I did not want to do anything. I did not even long for food or sweets. I didn't want to meet with anybody. I didn't even have the strength to pray. The only thing I wanted to do was sleep.

During our tour in the United States I had bought myself an English Bible. The contents were divided up as usual into books, epistles and chapters, but this edition was also divided up according to the calendar. The idea was that one should read a little every day and thus read through the Bible in one year. Even though I felt really awful, I got hold of that book and started to read.

It was not exactly anything new to me. It was the same story of creation as in other Bibles that I had read many times, the same slavery in Egypt, the same, the same. . . .

After a few days of rest, however, I noticed how the old joy and zest for life started to come back, and I thought I felt particularly well during the times when I was reading my English Bible.

I was soon a lot better, but now I had to sit down and think things through properly. During the last few years my whole life had been directed by the two words "if only" and "then." When life was all work during my training in swimming, I had thought: "If only *I were allowed to give myself to singing properly* — then *everything will become much easier.*" And then later, when I was right in the middle of my music studies, I had thought, "If only *I could finish college and be allowed to sing full-time* — then *my whole existence will become much better.*"

Now I was a full-time singer, but I had banged my head against the wall just the same.

At the same time I was thinking through my motives—and God's.

My parents had always encouraged me to follow my heart: to do that which felt right in the innermost part of my being. All my life my longing had been to do that which God wanted me to do. I knew that everything would turn out for the best then.

But now I began to question whether I was still following my heart. Perhaps I was just singing because now everybody wanted to hear me sing. I no longer enjoyed performing and holding concerts. The only thing I wanted to do, and the only thing I could do just then, was to listen to my innermost being again.

I didn't suddenly stop singing — not least because the pressure was on from Japan and I had promised to make a long tour during the spring of 1992. But I felt fairly soon that I needed a break in order to think over what I wanted to do with my life from now on. I decided to go to Bible School.

This was how I got to India!

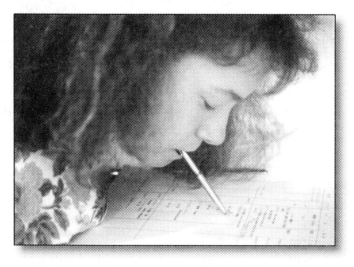

I am a person who perseveres and looks at life positively.

12

What I Learned in India

I wake because my forehead is itching. That will be yet another mosquito bite then. It is dark and cold, I am feeling sick and am terribly tired, but I am not able to go back to sleep. Everything is quiet except for the breathing of the two girls who are sharing the same room with me.

A mosquito comes whining, but disappears again while I lie there thinking.

If I had known what it would be like to live here in India, I don't know if I would have come. Everything is so different—and dirty. A couple of days ago I tried to put on a little perfume, but five minutes later I could not smell its fragrance. Now I have become accustomed *to all the odors. But when we landed and stepped out of the plane, we were met by an indescribably bad smell.*

Now I am lying here awake early in the morning on this first day of the New Year. Imagine starting a new year this way, in a sleeping bag sixty-five hundred kilometers from home! I am completely dried out in the mouth, for I have developed a sinus infection. And at the same time it feels as if my whole body is itching, and I don't think it is just bites from mosquitoes. I have developed a strange eczema on my chin and cheek, which I have never had before, and I look terrible. I have now been lying on this bed for more than three days and three nights, except for when I have been running to the toilet because of diarrhea. . . .

So I was in Karnal.

After three months' studies in an international Bible School in Amsterdam together with forty students from many different countries, we all went to India to practice what we had learned. Five of my classmates and I were to go to Karnal, a few hours' journey by bus north of New Delhi in order to work together with Pastor Lal and his small church. We lived together with the pastor and his family in a tiny house and helped with the services. These were held in his garage, which had been made into a church.

We were three girls who shared a room in which we only just had room for our beds, but for absolutely nothing else. It was crowded everywhere. Wherever one turned around in this house one bumped against somebody else. On top of all this, people in the village had heard about the visiting foreigners, so many people came to visit. I, who had lived alone on eighty square meters in Stockholm and been able to freely dispose of my time, found it very hard to get used to things.

For example, I wanted to go out in the street by myself, but this was impossible, for it was considered dangerous. Especially for a woman. If anyone needed to go to the post office or bank, somebody else always had to accompany this person, and it could sometimes take half a day. We therefore needed to plan almost every day in detail and learn to adjust six different and strong wills.

To be a woman in India was not the way it was at home. We were treated quite differently here, and all of us girls were forced to consider our behavior. We had to make sure we never looked a man in the eye, for this could have unexpected consequences.

My situation as a disabled person, however, was probably the most difficult to handle. For the first time in my life, I *felt* that I was handicapped. At home I was used to handling everything myself. I had always lived like everybody else and had hardly ever experienced my lack of arms as a great hindrance. Naturally I do things in a different way, but my disability had almost never limited what I had wanted to do.

In India there were so many things I couldn't do. All the time I was forced to ask for help, and this was something I had never needed to do before—at least not to this extent. I felt as if I was being taken care of against my will. It was hard not to be able to help with either the cooking or the washing up. I could not shower by myself, and going to the toilet was often problematic.

And yet it felt as if God was with me. So, for instance, ours was the only team that had Western-style toilets everywhere, and I was so grateful for this. But, of course, the toilets did not always flush when we wanted them to, and this could naturally cause problems. Filling a tin bucket to the brim and then pouring it in the toilet was too heavy a job for me, so on such occasions I always had to ask for help.

But on one occasion when I was the victim of a tummy upset and had been to the toilet for the umpteenth time, I really didn't feel like opening the door for anyone, for the smell which would then spread from there was not exactly pleasant. I stood there, very irritably wondering if I might be able to solve the problem without asking for help. I then came to think of all those fantastic stories which missionaries had told us during my childhood, about how they had prayed to God in emergency situations and seen all kinds of things happening. Well, this clearly was a kind of emergency situation!

So before I had time to really grasp what I was doing, I said in a loud and determined voice:

"Work, in the Name of Jesus!"

I pulled the lever—and suddenly it flushed as never before. I could hardly believe my eyes!

This became the thing which other people in the

house also did on visits to the toilet, and even if it did not work every time, it was fun when it did. I also believe that it was episodes like this one that enabled me to cope with my months in India.

The following incident is another example of this:

It so happened that soon after we had arrived in India I had to leave my class for a week because I had promised to fly to Japan to sing at an event which the United Nations had arranged. I came back to Bombay where my classmates were just then, but something appeared to be wrong. We landed in the middle of the night, and the airport was crowded with people.

I tried to ask an Indian man who was helping me with my bags what was wrong, but he did not understand what I was saying. It looked as if I wouldn't be able to leave the airport. Gradually I got to know that all the bus and taxi services had stopped running and that I could not leave the airport.

However, a pilot helped me to get up to a departure lounge where I would be allowed to stay the night. Several times guards came and drove out everybody else, but I was allowed to remain sitting there.

Near to five o'clock in the morning I asked one of the guards if I could possibly get a taxi, but the only thing he answered was:

"Dangerous, dangerous!"

And later when I asked him again, he said:

"Still dangerous!"

When it became light, he asked me to follow him. He said that even though it was still dangerous, this would be the best time to leave. I was allowed out through a back door where a taxi was waiting. The taxi driver wanted twice the normal fare and half of the amount in advance. I just wanted to leave, so I gave him what he wanted, and he drove away at a mad speed into the city.

It was frightening to find all the streets deserted. Where two weeks earlier the pavements had been crowded with people who lived there, it was now empty. The nearer we came to the city, the more careful his driving became. At every crossroads he stopped and looked very carefully before he pressed the accelerator to the boards until he got to the next block.

A policeman who wanted a lift was allowed to jump in, while the taxi driver drove farther and farther. Why weren't there any people about? Why was it dangerous? Why did it take so long to arrive at our destination? I became more and more scared. I don't think I have ever prayed so intensely to God, either before or after this event.

When at last we stopped in front of the youth hostel where my classmates were staying, I got out of the taxi on trembling legs and walked in. I was told that there had been a four-day curfew in Bombay because there had been fighting between Muslims and Hindus, so my taxi journey could have finished badly. I felt relieved to have arrived at my destination and so grateful to God for his protection through it all.

Even though my time in India was the most difficult time I have ever experienced, it did shape me and my way of thinking very much. My faith became deeper, and I learned to appreciate things that I had never really valued before. My desire for music returned, and I felt motivated to start singing in earnest again.

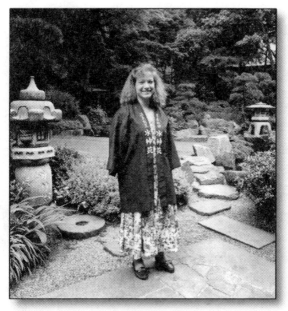

I love Japan.

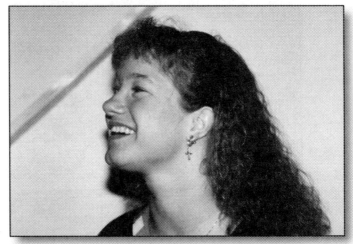

It was tough when I was in India,
but I felt again that I should sing.

13

Sayonara—
Japan in
My Heart

J apan will always have a big place in my heart.

When I visited Japan for the first time after the two films about me had been shown, and after I had been interviewed on television, I was not able to imagine what an impact it would all make. I just liked to be interviewed and liked to sing in a live broadcast.

In both of the two earlier television reports, for very understandable reasons, everything I had said about my faith, and about God, had been deleted before the broadcasts. Seeing that there are so many religions in Japan, the policy which television has adopted, generally speaking, is never to bring up people's philosophy of life in their programs. But now when the presenter of the *News Station* program asked me why I seemed to be so happy and had the strength to do so much, I could not help but tell him about my faith.

Now everybody got to know that I was a Christian, and immediately representatives of various churches started to get in touch to ask me to come and sing. One of them was Alf Idland, a Norwegian clergyman working in Kobe who had lived in Japan for almost twenty years. He arranged a tour of just over two weeks for Anders and me in May 1992. He became my manager.

Churches in different places backed the concerts, but not everybody was as convinced as Alf about how great the interest was for this Swedish vocalist who, in spite of everything, was still fairly unknown. When, in the city of Mishima, Bo Dellming, a Swedish missionary, rented the biggest concert hall for our concert, which could hold around twelve hundred people. His church would not back this venture, so he had to rent the hall at his own risk. However, he did not have to worry for very long, for we had so many people coming that evening that we had to give an extra performance the same evening.

It was fantastic! All the concerts were sold out, and on many occasions so much so that it was standing room only. There were long queues outside the concert halls for several hours beforehand. People whom we did not know came up to us asking for autographs. Anders and I were completely taken aback, but I slowly started to grasp what an impact the TV programs had made.

The Japanese liked my singing and the beautiful, sometimes slightly sad tunes that I presented, but this was not the only reason why they came to the concerts.

Through the TV programs, many Japanese people had been given a picture of a disabled person which was different from the picture they were otherwise used to. The following excerpt is an example of this. It is from the *Yomiuri* newspaper in Japan in which a TV journalist commented on one of the films about me:

On 19 June in the evening programme News Station *we saw a video film about Lena Maria*

*from Sweden who is studying at a music con-
servatory to become a singer. . . . This video film
really showed that the worth of a human being
is in her soul.*

And then the reporter gave a few other examples of
the same thing:

*In a shop in Hawaii there was a girl who was
asked something. The girl was disabled because
of thalidomide, but she showed the way with her
small hands. In another shop there was a young
man who was dumb, but a sign had been put up
asking people to put their money on the counter.*

*If we behave in a normal way and help these
people, they too will be enabled to do as much as
their ability allows. We know that even people
without handicaps are better at doing some things
than other things. I have discovered that overseas
people see these things and feel it is wonderful,
whereas I notice that we Japanese do not have as
much sympathy.* (From the Yomiuri newspaper)

Well, I think they may have sympathy, but in Japan it is considered a great shame to have a handicapped child. The shame is so great that the parents hide the children or give them away, and it can be difficult even for somebody who is the brother or sister of a handicapped person to get married. Few disabled persons go to school. Most of them live in institutions and occupy themselves by baking, sewing or manufacturing various things that they can sell. For a disabled person to go to college and live an independent life like I do is something tremendous in the eyes of the Japanese.

The Japanese are brought up to succeed. This is true from the time they are small and have to learn to handle the competitive situation at school, until they are grown up and must succeed at work. It is also true about Japan as a nation. People are incredibly efficient in their pursuit of the key to success. They might travel the world over in order to obtain tips and ideas on how to become even more efficient and successful. They often succeed in their pursuit, and many times Japanese products are on top in the world market.

In this way of life probably lies something of the explanation as to why the Japanese were fascinated—and still continue to be fascinated—by me, for in their eyes I have succeeded. I am living a life which is just about impossible for a severely disabled person. Japanese people want to know what lies behind my successes. These questions keep coming back all the time when I am interviewed by journalists or when I meet ordinary people in the street.

It was not just through our tour that we knew the interest was great. A Japanese record company also showed their interest at an early stage. They made sure that the CD that Anders and I had already recorded in English was printed with a Japanese cover, and soon this company wanted us to make a new recording.

For our first CD, Anders and I had quite a small budget, but this second one really became a large production. Approximately sixty musicians took part with violins, wind instruments, percussion instruments, guitar, bass, key harp and a lot of other instruments and effects. Anders and I even went to Hollywood and recorded a few songs together with guitarist Larry Carlton, and percussionist Alex Acuña. I wrote several songs myself, or together with Anders, for this music production which received the title *My Life*.

Then *My Life* became a book. It was written by a Japanese author who was in Sweden interviewing me for one week through an interpreter. But as if this were not enough, another two books were made: one about my parents and their views of the disabled person, and also a schoolbook for primary-school children. In Japan, children are given a book as an assignment for them to read over the summer holidays. It is a book about which they must write an essay, and my book was chosen in several of the Japanese school districts for this purpose. In addition, a small booklet was published in English and was used in English classes in schools.

When occasionally I pull out all these books with their beautiful full-color pictures of me and my family, but written with characters which I do not understand at all, and with their front page on the back page so to say, it naturally does feel quite remarkable.

At the time of this writing, I have done six different kinds of tours in Japan, both long and short. Occasionally I tour just with Anders; on other occasions I perform with a trio or a symphony orchestra. Usually, there have been quite big arrangements with many people involved. During one of the tours in 1995 when I sang together with Anders Wihk's jazz trio we had forty people with us who looked after the sound, lighting and stage. That is as big as the Rock Train, the biggest concert tour that runs every summer in Sweden, said the filmmakers, Sven-Eric Frick and Henrik Burman, when they were in Japan during the tour.

But during the tour something very sad happened. Alf Idland, our manager, became sick with cancer. Because he knew that he would not be able to cope with the full role of being manager, he had handed over the responsibility to other people at an early stage, and only came to visit us now and then. He appeared to be quite well anyway, and it looked as if he would be able to conquer his sickness.

However, this was not to be the case. The sickness got the better of him, and he died in his sleep at the peak of

the tour. This was very sad news. We cancelled the concerts for two days to attend his funeral. It was hard to
lose Alf, both as a friend and as our manager.

And now what would become of our future tours? It
felt uncertain for a while, but when we asked our friend,
Katsutada Sugitani, we were fairly soon given a positive
answer. He had often been an adviser to Alf Idland, and
so was comparatively well-versed in what was happening. He took over as manager and has helped us incredibly since then.

Their interest in me seems to last. It is always enjoyable to receive attention, but at the same time it is
demanding. All the time I am being watched, so I must
think carefully about what I do and how I perform. It
feels like being in public all day and all night sometimes.
Besides, it is difficult to really get to know people in
depth.

Sometimes I have actually thought of moving to this
"empire of the sun," but I don't think it would work in
the long run. Nevertheless, Japan has a special place in
my heart. I believe I have been able to give many people

a new attitude toward the disabled, and perhaps I have also been able to give them an understanding of what the Christian faith is all about. At the same time, I have learned an enormous amount myself, met interesting people and have had many enjoyable experiences.

Definitely the most enjoyable, and the most different, experience I have had was for television—together with Santa Claus in Sweden!

It was after the big earthquake in Kobe that the TV channel Asahi got in touch, wanting me to participate in a program which was going to be aired over Christmas. During one of my tours I accompanied the TV team visiting some of the people who were living in the part of Kobe that had been hardest hit. I visited a temporary tent church which was held up by enormous cardboard tubes. I was interviewed and asked to sing with the children there for a TV special for Christmas 1995.

But the children of Kobe had more contact with Sweden. During the year, a school class in Sweden had made lots of drawings, which they had sent to the children in Kobe. This was the reason why Miss Sweden, together with the director of the Swedish "Tomteland" (Santa's Land), went to Kobe to deliver the drawings.

On December twenty-second, I travelled to "Tomteland" just outside Mora in the province of Dalarna (Darlicarlia), in order to be part of a technologically advanced TV show. In this program, which is one of the most popular programs in Japan and was being broadcast live, I got to tell the Japanese children about the place which I was visiting, and simultaneously a lady in the TV studio in Japan interpreted me.

As the next part of the program, they showed a report about my visit to Kobe and the handing over of the drawings. But then came the most exciting part. I sang "Silent Night" standing outside, in the snow, in the Darlicarlia forest while I (or rather my voice via satellite) was being accompanied by a pianist who was sitting in Kobe.

Because of the time it takes for sound to travel between Asia and Europe, in spite of the advances that science has made, I was not able to listen to his piano accompaniment, so he had to merely accompany my song. We never had time to practice together, so it was a little nerve-wracking. It just had to work in the live broadcast.

Everything went superbly, but I have never, before or after, been part of anything like it.

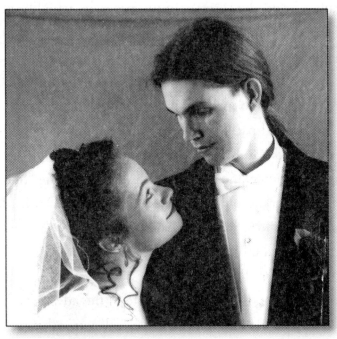

Björn and I

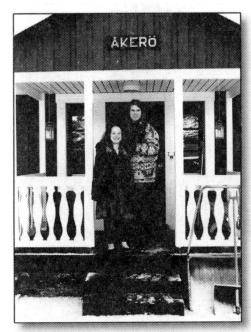

Björn and I in front of a previous home

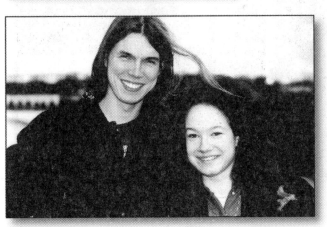

I am glad to have Björn's help when there are problems.

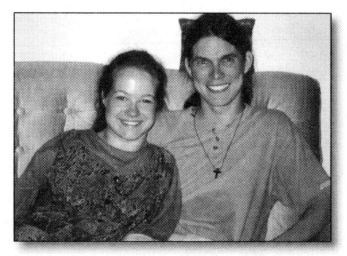

At home

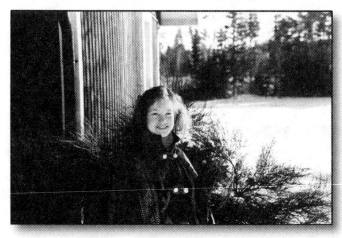

Me, in front of the house

14

We Were
Just
Friends

Can one have a relationship when one is as disabled as I am? If one is to get married, ought one not marry somebody who is as disabled as oneself? Besides, are there any guys at all who are interested?

It seems that many people have wondered about this, and many have asked me if I would like to get married and start a family. But, as with so many other things, I have not thought a great deal about it. I have kind of handed it over to God, for he has arranged so many other things in my life.

Naturally, I have sometimes longed very much for a

man. What girl does not do this in her teens and early twenties? Many times I have been in love and thought that *now* it must be right, here is the man in my life, but then it hasn't worked out.

Then I met Björn.

We got to know each other through the gospel choir called The Master's Voice at the Music Conservatory. I was one of the cofounders of the choir, and when we had our first concert several people wanted to join us. Björn Klingvall, who was studying to become a music teacher and whose main instrument was viola, wanted to join us to sing tenor. We immediately found that we had a lot in common.

We started to meet now and then to have lunch together and to talk about whatever was close to our hearts at the time. Björn became the kind of friend I could talk with about everything. A real brother! I think he felt that he could talk about quite a number of things with me, too, for when he had girlfriend problems he came to me.

It may sound like a cliché, but we were just friends,

and to me this was something natural. There were so many things which indicated that we could not become a couple. I understood that it was quite important to Björn how girls looked on the outside. To me, it was important that the one with whom I would eventually share my life would also share my faith. Besides, we were not at all in love, at least not with each other.

Even though Björn did not consider himself to be a Christian, we still talked a lot about God. This was quite natural since he was also a member of the choir, but after a while he left. He felt it was too tough when everybody was talking about their faith and Jesus, and it was too stressful to sing about these things which he did not know if he believed in.

I felt bad for his sake, and I prayed for him, for I knew that he was having a tough time, but we did not meet each other as often anymore. For a while, when, among other things, I was on a tour in the United States, we lost contact altogether, but I continued to send up little prayers for him.

When I came back to Sweden I went to choir

practice with The Master's Voice, and there, to my great surprise, I found Björn. He told me that he had just woken up one day and felt that there had to be a God after all, and that all those things about Jesus were probably true. Now he felt that he could sing gospel and really mean what he was singing. That's why he had started to sing in the choir again.

During the spring, we continued to meet more and more frequently. We tried to see what it was like to go on the motorbike together, we listened to music together, we talked, we went to concerts and a lot of other things. In the summer, we even went on holiday together on the motorbike.

We were like the best of friends, but we still did not have any thought about "getting together" with each other. To be married to Björn would feel like having a relationship with one's own brother! When people asked us if we were a couple, we just laughed. I had a fantastic friend, and that was enough.

The months passed, however, and gradually there

was a question which started to buzz around inside me: What would life with Björn be like?

"No, it would never work," I said to myself.

The question continued to buzz, but I knew the answer as firmly each time. Of course it was fantastic that he was a believer, but he was not at all the type of man I had dreamed of marrying. Besides, I could see several things which meant that a relationship between us would not work. For instance, he would have to be able to help me without my asking him every time, for it would never work otherwise.

And then the miracle happened. Björn started to change.

It started one evening when I came home from a tour. That's when he treated me to the evening meal. He had never done this before. And the following morning he came over to my flat and cooked breakfast. And then he washed up!

It was as if every time I mentioned to God which things would not work, Björn started to change in this area. It was remarkable. At the same time, I started to seriously wonder if I would be able to love Björn through my whole life as my husband. Well, this was something one could never really know, could one? But after some time I knew that if Björn ever proposed to me, my answer would be "yes."

I had never felt my disability was a hindrance in any way, except when it came to this matter. I felt that I could not take the first step and talk about the possibility of a future together. I did know that it is quite demanding to be married to a disabled person, and on top of this my unusual work did not exactly make things easier. Least of all did I want Björn to feel pressured. I wanted his choice, if he were to choose me, to come from within himself.

But now I was really in love.

I was scheduled to go to Japan on a tour again when Björn brought up the subject that I most of all wanted to talk about. Oh yes, he had also been thinking about us and our relationship, he told me, and together we decided to think the whole thing over while we were separated—he in Sweden and I in Japan. We decided that if we both felt as if we wanted to continue with our relationship, we would get engaged in time for Christmas.

For my part I saw it as an ultimatum: I wanted a whole-hearted "yes" from Björn if he were to choose me. The three-week tour in Japan felt terribly long. I myself knew what I wanted, so emotionally I was thrown between hope and despair. Anders, my poor pianist, had to devote time to advanced counseling between the concerts.

For Björn, it was not easy. He was really my friend, but could he think of me as his woman and his wife? Also, was he prepared to live with my handicap?

At last the weeks in Japan were over. It was one week before Christmas, and I landed at Arlanda Airport where Björn stood waiting.

I received a welcoming hug, but I was very nervous before I was told what decision he had reached. Did he love me, or didn't he? It was a lot worse than when you pull the petals off a daisy!

I asked him about it in the car as we were leaving the airport.

Yes, he did love me! He had decided to share his whole life with me, and to both of us it felt as if this was also something God wanted.

Two days before Christmas, we were engaged at a wonderful little inn outside Vadstena. You may think that this is incredible, but I received my first kiss at the same time that we exchanged rings. The whole evening was fantastic, and on the way to the inn we experienced a sunset that was just as fantastic. It was as if God was smiling on us.

Our engagement was no testing period. We had made our decision. The following spring months, therefore, went very quickly since we had to prepare for our wedding and all that this entailed.

Because we both knew so many people but didn't have so many close friends, we hesitated a little concerning whether to have a big or a small wedding. We chose to have a big wedding, but at the same time we chose to say "no, thank you" to most of the mass media that were lining up to see our wedding. Even though I was a well-known person, we did not want our wedding day to be primarily a TV film.

And so, on July 1, 1995, we were married in the Gustav Wasa Church in Stockholm with more than eight hundred guests present as witnesses. When I was younger it had been my dream that my wedding would also become a concert— and this really did happen. We did know that The Master's Voice was going to sing Handel's "Messiah" as the recessional, but in addition Marina Johansson, our good friend who organized the wedding, had arranged several musical surprises in the form of a concert which lasted for half an hour.

The following day we went on our honeymoon by motorbike through Europe. When we came home we had seven thousand kilometers behind us.

I had found the husband who was the very best, and the one who had been my very best friend ever. He is the finest person I know and has a wonderful and warm heart. I was happy on that day, and I am still happy, proud and thankful for finding Björn of all people.

This does not mean that everything since then has been cozy fairy-tale happiness. Some illusions have already disappeared. For instance, we thought that we knew each other so terribly well before we married, and in a way we were indeed very close friends, but I discovered that I had been carrying things inside which I had never shared with anybody.

Naturally, we have had to go through the same things as most newlyweds, but to live with a disability is sometimes more difficult after one has married. It can have to do with both small and big things: from knowing how much help I need, or do not need, in order for the marriage to work in the best possible way, to how we show tenderness towards one another. To sit "foot in hand" with Björn is an example of what feels natural for me but does not feel natural for Björn.

It is fortunate that we can often find a solution by talking with each other. We never put the lid on our problems, and we have learned to turn to God even more than before.

15

You Saw
Me Before I
Was Born

Thank you that you exist. . . . But I think that if you had been an average "Svensson" you might have been sitting in a wheel-chair in an institution.

What a zest for life you have! It is fantastic to see how much you are able to do. But how can you manage to pull up a pair of trousers, and how can you button up all the buttons everywhere? . . . I'm sure you must have some-body helping you with these.

I receive many letters from people, both in Japan and in Sweden. Often they wonder how I can have such a positive outlook on life all the time, and how I have succeeded in so many things, in spite of the odds that were against me.

This is a hard question, but I think I can see at least three different reasons. First, it is quite simply so, isn't it, that when we are born we are all different? I was happy and curious about life from the start. My personality is such that I would look at the possibilities rather than the difficulties. I do not make things more difficult than they are. I think positively about myself. I dare to help myself to things I see. I dare to ask.

I am stubborn. My disability has encouraged this stubbornness in a good way. I think that if I had an ordinary body, my stubbornness and positive thinking would have made me self-centered and would have resulted in my elbowing myself forward in life. My disability has instead helped me not to take everything for granted.

The second reason is my parents. Their relaxed attitude toward me and my disability has been incredibly important. They have given me a very secure foundation. They have helped me to succeed, as well as to accept failure. They have propped me up, but they have never made my handicap more important than my person. Of course they have often had to tell people about my lack of mobility and so on, but they did not let the conversation revolve around me.

I think the third, and most important, reason why I have always had such a happy outlook on life is undoubtedly God. Faith has been such a natural part of my life for as long as I can remember, and as a Christian I know that I have worth whoever I am and however I look.

I often think of a few Scripture verses from Psalm 139:

> *You created my inmost being; you knit me together in my mother's womb. I praise you because I am fearfully and wonderfully made; your works are wonderful, I know that full well. My frame was not hidden from you when I was made in the secret place. When I was woven in the depths of the earth, your eyes saw my unformed*

body. All the days ordained for me were written
in your book before one of them came to be.

Was God with me already at the fetus stage? Did he think of me before I was born? Yes, I believe this, and I also believe that to him it is not my looks and my shape that are most important. The most important thing of all is my relationship with him. I know that he loves me.

Of course I have wondered many times why there is so much suffering and trouble, sicknesses and disabilities, and there are times when I have wondered how God can allow such things. Not that I have any easy solutions, but perhaps it is so because it is precisely the things that hurt us that shape us as human beings. Perhaps darkness must exist in order to enhance the light.

No human being goes through life without problems, but the richness of being a human being is something which I believe one comes to realize, first of all, through difficult experiences. I notice this when I meet people whom I admire. It is their way of coping with difficulties in life which makes them so admirable.

A person I admire very much is Aiako Miura,* the Japanese author who lives on Hokkaido, an island in northern Japan. Throughout her life she has been suffering from various illnesses which have been almost too much for her. But in some way or other she has always managed to get through the difficulties, and they have given her strength. In Japan, she is a great Christian author, and her books have meant a lot to many people. She has written over seventy books during her lifetime, more than thirty million copies have been sold, and several of her books have been translated into other languages.

She keeps on writing, although she is now old and suffering from both Parkinson's disease and cancer. I met her and her husband during one of my visits to Japan, and this was both enjoyable and instructive. Their courage, joy and warmth made a strong impression on me.

When comparing myself to people like these I do not think that I have had a particularly difficult time in life. God has given me the strength to cope with what pain

*Aiako Miura died in October 1999.

and suffering I have had to go through, and I am only glad if my life — with all its ups and downs — can mean anything for another human being.

Naturally, I have sometimes wished that God would heal me. I never thought like this when I was younger, but I do so from time to time nowadays. I feel that my body is becoming stiffer, and my hips ache easily when there is too much weight on them. It would be practical to have arms. It would make it easier. And it would be a miracle!

But I see it as a miracle that I am privileged to have God with me even in the way I look today. I agree with Joni Eareckson Tada, an American woman who was paralyzed through a diving accident, whom I heard saying about her handicap and her faith something like this: "If God were to act and heal me I would be happy. But to be able to live happily in the midst of a difficult situation, this shows even more how great God is."

Some people may think that my faith is naïve, but I have seen so many times that God has been with me in both big and small situations. This gives me joy and energy. That's why I can also continue to look positively towards the future, even though I do not know a great deal about what is going to happen. I am glad to be alive and to be a singer. I have a husband, family and friends who can help me when life is difficult. But, above all, I have God. He loves me, and I know that nothing can take this love from me.

When I participated in the Paralympic Games in Seoul, Korea, I wrote a song about how it felt to travel alone. I would like to share the words with you:

Somewhere inside me I can hear You whispering my name
As a wind, quietly whispering
You are there.
I am resting in Your arms,
You are saying to me that You love me
and that You want to be my very best friend.
Just imagine that
wherever I am, You are always there.
You care about my innermost being
and You take time to ask how I am.
You know about everything which I cannot understand,

All my faults, but You love me anyway,
You love me, You love me anyway.

Postscript

I t's been more than five years since the first edition of *Footnotes* was published in Sweden. Of course, many things have happened since then.

In 1997, I took a year off from all my travelling and singing. I also got the chance to start painting again, which I hope I'll have time to develop in the future. A new album—together with the Swedish Radio Symphony Orchestra—became a reality during 1998.

The Japanese people don't seem to get tired of me, so I have continued to go there two to three times a year. I had the privilege of singing at the opening ceremony of the Paralympic Games in Nagano, and my pianist, Anders Wihk, and I also gave a concert at the Zenkoji Temple. I didn't know anyone could sing and talk about Jesus in a Buddhist Temple, but it went really well!

Thailand also shows a great interest in my work now, and I have just visited and been singing with Princess Chulaborn of Thailand. Concerts in Korea and Taiwan are also planned for the future.

My husband and I have moved from the countryside and are back in Stockholm. People are wondering if we have any children yet, but that has to wait for a little while longer.

Since its original publication in Sweden, my book has been translated to Norwegian, Danish, Finnish, German, French, Thai, Japanese, Estonian and English. It's a great joy for me that *Footnotes* continues to live on.